THE GIFT OF PASSIONARIES™

May these profiles ignite
your own passions. You can
create ripples.
                    Enjoy!
                        Barbara Metzler

Passionaries Press
Suite 108A #425
Carlsbad Village Drive
Carlsbad, CA 92008-2999
Fax: (760) 757-1855

Most of *The Gift of Passionaries*' profiles have involved personal telephone interviews with information updated through each nonprofit's web site listed at the end of each profile. Stories included in this book were collected over a period of 7 years. Reasonable care has been taken to trace original ownership and, when necessary, to obtain permission to print or reprint. If the author has overlooked giving proper credit to anyone, please contact Passionaries LLC at the address above.

Book designed and typeset by Teresa Haymaker

Cover designed by: Jan Funchess, Teresa Haymaker, and Rodney Bissell

Metzler, Barbara R.
    The gift of passionaries changing our world : how can I turn
    compassion into action? / Barbara R. Metzler. — 1st ed. — Carlsbad,
    CA : Passionaries Press, c2008.
        p. ; cm.
        (Passionaries: turning compassion into action)
        ISBN: 978-0-9821776-0-0
        Includes bibliographical references and index.
    1. Compassion—Case studies. 2. Social entrepreneurship—Case
    studies. 3. Voluntarism—Case studies. 4. Volunteers—Case studies.
    I. Title.

BJ1475 .M484 2008   2008938899
361.7092/273—dc22   0810

Printed in the United States of America
First Edition, 2009

PASSIONARIES™ is a trademark and service mark of Barbara Metzler.

The Gift

of PASSIONARIES™
CHANGING OUR WORLD

How can I turn
compassion into action?

Barbara R. Metzler

Table of Contents

Preface

Since this is the second in a series of Passionaries Institute books, you might be interested to know how it came about. A few years back, I retired from being a serial entrepreneur and moved with my family from Fresno to San Diego, California, wanting to enjoy my last two children as they completed high school. Facing an empty nest, I prayed about what God wanted me to do in the next season my life.

Shortly thereafter, I attended a World Presidents Organization meeting where a prize-winning environmentalist challenged the audience to "Do whatever you can to change television." He was from the Caribbean island of Dominica and was talking about how America is viewed by foreigners as a violent and dangerous place due to the television shows and news. With that challenge, my life changed.

After this meeting, I could not sleep for three nights. I knew God was speaking to me through that man. The change in my life was dramatic. I was an entrepreneur who shunned publicity. Now as an author and speaker, I seek positive media exposure to tip the broadcast scale, balancing the dire with the inspired.

It seems as though the vast majority of media is convinced that "it needs to bleed to lead." Are they right? Is that the only world you want to know? Is that the image we want to share with those abroad? Does the media project a balanced reality of the world in which you live? If you believe all that you hear and read, we live in a Gotham of darkness with just occasional glimpses of light, and no Batman in sight.

I am convinced that the difference between darkness and light can be as simple as the flip of a switch, like an inspiring story that causes a paradigm shift. You control the switch on how you perceive the world: Let there be light!

As the writer who coined the word *passionaries*, my calling is to collect and share real stories of courage and greatness. I count it a privilege and a pleasure. I invite you to join me in this mission. The health of our country and the world may hinge on our collective will to get these passionate visionaries and their organizations headlined in mainstream media. Millions of times in millions of ways every day, individuals turn their compassion into action, usually unnoticed and unacknowledged. This benevolent spirit is the legacy of our great country.

For every problem faced, there are multiple problem-solvers, knights in shining armor—they are every day people, humanitarians. Those profiled in this book reflect a small sampling of the unsung real-life heroes fighting for truth, justice and the American way—just as the mythical Superman did in comic books. Their stories are classically riveting, with each real individual tackling tremendous odds to make a difference for others whose names they may never know. In reading of the passionaries' struggles and successes, you will receive a gift of insight and hope that can brighten reality and stir your own passions.

Gifts come in many shapes, forms, and sizes. They are a blessing of love for both the receiver and giver, bringing deep, lasting joy. One of the favorite gifts I've ever received is a cheery little pink box with a white bow that my daughter gave me. The note on it says: "This present is not to be opened. It is filled with my love for you. And it is to be a constant reminder that someone cares enough for you to give you a gift of love. Whenever the world gets you down, think of this gift and you will never frown." It has remained unopened for 25 years, and I cherish it dearly.

This book is filled with gifts for you to cherish. The stories celebrate the contributions that passionaries make toward solving social problems and helping people in need. To all of you who are passionaries, passioneers (volunteers), and passionors (donors): *thank you for your gifts.* You embody the power of your name: *Amer-I-Can.* Ripples of goodness emanate from your compassionate actions. You change our world.

If you have ever wondered how to turn compassion into action, you are reading the perfect book! In the introduction, you will learn the incredible facts of American giving and volunteering, followed by inspiring purpose-driven profiles and the ripples they create. In the "Engage and Empower" pages, discover how *you* can take action, and connect with marvelous resources for community change. My promise to you is that when you have read about all the role models spotlighted in this book, you will know unequivocally the answer to three significant questions:

- ♥ Can any one person change our world?
- ♥ Just how great are Americans at giving and volunteering?
- ♥ What ripples are created by giving to others?

Before Passionaries, you might have thought, "There is so much bad news, I don't even watch the news anymore. There is nothing I can do to make a difference. The problem is just too big. It's beyond me."

Please hear me. That's not true. You can make a difference. There is a lot you can do. Beware that by reading this book, your own passions may be ignited. Discovering the incredible gifts of these passionaries could shift your worldview to one of positive optimism. You can empower others, leaving wondrous ripples of transformed lives in your wake.

Enjoy and savor the passionaries and their nonprofits in this book, then go forth and passionate!

—*Barbara Metzler*

P.S. This is my favorite song because it epitomizes the passionary heart. May we all be like Don Quixote, the Man of La Mancha, on a quest and dreaming the impossible dream.

THE IMPOSSIBLE DREAM
Lyrics by Joe Darion, Music by Mitch Leigh

To dream the impossible dream, to fight the unbeatable foe,
To bear with unbearable sorrow, to run where the brave dare not go.

To right the unrightable wrong, to love pure and chaste from afar,
to try when your arms are too weary, to reach the unreachable star.

This is my quest, to follow that star-
no matter how hopeless, no matter how far.

To fight for the right without question or pause,
to be willing to march into hell for a heavenly cause.

And I know if I'll only be true to this glorious quest
That my heart will be peaceful and calm, when I'm laid to my rest.

And the world will be better for this,
That one man scorned and covered with scars,

Still strove with his last ounce of courage,
to reach the unreachable stars.

Dedication

A country like the United States is conducive to producing passionary citizens like the ones profiled in *The Gift of Passionaries*. This book is offered in honor of all the nonprofit passionaries, their volunteers, and donors who together create greatness. Your efforts are not always acknowledged, yet your vision touches and inspires and your actions ripple out, transforming untold numbers of lives. Thank you for the gift you give in serving humanity.

This book is dedicated to my God, with thanks for your gentle nudgings and minor miracles that keep me pointed in a positive direction. Thank you for giving us a country that is free, where "giving forward" is both our legacy and our promise. May you continue to bless and watch over America—and bless those who give. With all my love, I also dedicate this book to my amazing family.

Previous book by Barbara R. Metzler:
Passionaries: Turning Compassion into Action,
published by Templeton Foundation Press,
October 2006.

THE GIFT OF PASSIONARIES™

Definitions

Passionary: \\'pash-e,ner-e\\ n (ca. 2005) 1. one inspired passionately through vision and compassion to actively change the world for the better: *visionary in action on a mission*; 2. society's agent of change: pioneer of benevolent innovation giving forward and causing positive ripples; 3. a social entrepreneur emboldened to make a difference, volunteering above and beyond responsibilities to family and work: *inspirational difference-maker*.

Passioneer: \\'pash-e-neer\\ n (ca. 2008) 1. a passionate volunteer, a transformational agent of social change, offering a service to help others of his own free will: *volunteer in action on a mission*; 2. one who renders service to others voluntarily above and beyond duty to family and work to help and aid others in need, requesting no financial consideration for actions given; 3. a person of compassion turning care for others into action requiring time, commitment and responsibility, generating lifechanging ripples.

Passionor: \\'pash-e-nor\\ n (ca. 2008) 1. one who passionately gives, donates or presents a financial gift: *a donor in action on a mission*; 2. a compassionate resource of human capital whose monetary gifts are intended to make a tangible difference for others in need; 3. an individual, corporate or foundation donor giving money with no expectation of financial return, generating ripples of social change.

Introduction

"Never doubt that a small group of thoughtful, committed citizens can change the world. Indeed, it's the only thing that ever has."

—Margaret Mead

Blink once, and you see all the headline-grabbing social problems in the news and your heart is heavy; you might feel discouraged and hopeless. Read this book and blink twice, and you will see the world differently, knowing that for every problem there are lots of problem-solvers *giving* and *living* the solutions. You'll feel the spine-tingling hope that ripples through people and nonprofit organizations you may have never even heard of, yet they create magic and miracles every day in every city and town across our country and around the globe. This book is filled with stories reflecting what is going *right* in our world.

Passionaries and their volunteers are *real* purpose-driven role models and heroes you can emulate and follow. Whether young or old, poor or wealthy, healthy or broken in body or soul, the models of passion in this book come in one color: radiant. Driven by a vision and a mission, they focus on positive possibilities. The sun shines brighter when your heart is ignited by passion to make a difference for others.

In simple terms, it takes three things to create a successful nonprofit organization: 1) *passionaries* with vision whose compassion ignites their call to action, 2) *passioneers* (volunteers) inspired to come alongside to turn dreams into reality, and 3) *passionors* (donors) who fund the solutions. What are the statistics on giving in the United States in these three areas of greatness? What does it take to be a passionary? And what does this all mean for you?

Hold on to your seats! This introduction explores these questions. You may never see Americans or yourself in the same way again.

Just How Great Are Americans At Giving?

Staggering, astounding, almost unbelievable generosity abounds in American hearts—generosity toward people in need, both in our country and around the world. The magnitude of U.S. giving and volunteering is in the *billions* of dollars each year. To understand the scope of giving, let's put the word 'billion' in a perspective we can understand. A billion is a 1 followed by nine zeroes (1,000,000,000). So 1 billion seconds ago—31.7 years—it was late 1975 and Richard Nixon had just left office, the Vietnam War ended, and pet rocks were cool. One billion minutes ago—a little more than 1,902 years—the Roman Empire ruled and the disciples of Jesus preached. A billion hours ago, we lived in the Stone Age.

Donors Giving Money

Before you read further, close your eyes and guess how much Americans gave to charity in 2006. It was in 1990 that charitable giving reached $100 billion. Despite three recessions since that date, giving has grown by huge amounts annually. Our donations to charity far surpass the economies of many countries. Americans in 2006 gave $295 *billion* to help those in need, almost tripling the record set in 1990.

Who gave the money and where it was directed are shown on the two charts below.

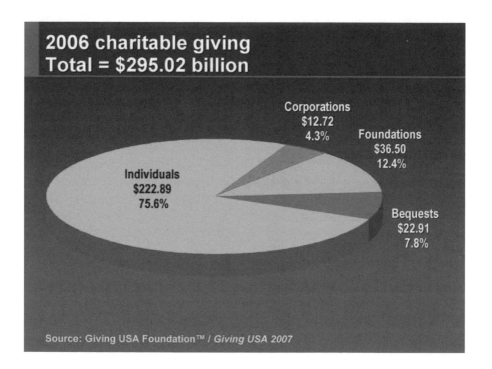

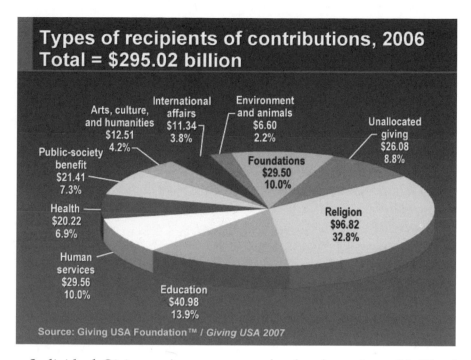

Types of recipients of contributions, 2006
Total = $295.02 billion

Arts, culture, and humanities $12.51 — 4.2%

International affairs $11.34 — 3.8%

Environment and animals $6.60 — 2.2%

Unallocated giving $26.08 — 8.8%

Public-society benefit $21.41 — 7.3%

Foundations $29.50 — 10.0%

Health $20.22 — 6.9%

Religion $96.82 — 32.8%

Human services $29.56 — 10.0%

Education $40.98 — 13.9%

Source: Giving USA Foundation™ / Giving USA 2007

Individual Giving ≈ As you can see by the above chart, 83.4% of all charitable giving comes from individuals, including gifts made by bequest. Many people believe the generous billionaires in our country give extraordinary amounts which account for most of this giving. Wrong. The Chronicles of Philanthropy studied the 50 most generous Americans for 2007 and found that collectively they gave $7.3 billion. As generous as that is, simple math shows that the vast majority of the magnificent $295 billion donated came from ordinary individuals who collectively made a huge difference. And we celebrate the awesome passionary billionaires. Six of the seven individuals who topped this prestigious list in 2007 were William Barron Hilton ($1.2 billion), Jon and Karen Huntsman ($750 million), T. Denny Sanford ($474 million), John Kluge ($400 million), Sanford and Joan Weill ($328 million), and Michael Bloomberg ($205 million).[2]

Foundation Giving ≈ The role of foundations in professionally directing grants is significant. In the past 10 years, their giving has increased by an average of 9.3% annually, adjusted for inflation. Donations by the country's 72,000 foundations hit a staggering new high of $36.5 billion in 2006, with overall assets of $614 billion. They are playing a progressively greater role in making grants, filling needs that are not covered by the government and which are closely overseen by trained foundation personnel.[3]

The trends show that some individual giving may be in the process of being replaced by individuals making gifts through family foundations, which accounts for half of the grant dollars awarded. From 2005–2006, giving by family foundations increased 13%, reaching a total of $16 billion, according to a report from the Foundation Center, a New York research group.[4] Their report identified 37,800 independent foundations with measurable donor or donor-family involvement. Giving while living is also a growing trend, with parents involving their children and grandchildren in creating philanthropic goals that will last.

In 2003, the most recent year for which data is available, the nation's 66,000 private charitable funds controlled an estimated $476 billion dollars. These foundations are changing the world in amazing ways. We take our hats off to the vital work of foundations, including the five wealthiest: Bill and Melinda Gates Foundation, Seattle, Washington ($29.1 billion), Ford Foundation, New York ($11.6 billion), Robert Wood Johnson Foundation, Princeton, New Jersey ($9 billion), Lilly Endowment, Inc., Indianapolis, Indiana ($8.3 billion), and W.K. Kellogg Foundation, Battle Creek, Michigan ($7.2 billion).[5]

Corporate Giving ≈ As every entrepreneur knows, the purpose of corporations is profit. When companies are profitable, employees are paid, bonuses are awarded, taxes are collected, and shareholders are happy. So it is remarkable that in 2006 corporations amassed profits and also donated an awesome $12.7 billion to charity.[6] This is hardly the image most people have of American corporate greed!

The Foundation Center analyzed 2,600-plus corporate foundations in 2006 that gave a record $4.2 billion, up 6% from the previous year. According to the Center, the top six corporate foundations that year were:

- ♥ Aventis Pharmaceuticals Health Care Foundation, Bridgewater, New Jersey: $217.8 million
- ♥ Bank of America Charitable Foundation, Charlotte, North Carolina: $200 million
- ♥ Citi Foundation, New York, New York: $137 million → global microfinance, finance education

- ♥ GE Foundation, Fairfield, Connecticut: $200+ million → education
- ♥ Target Foundation, St. Paul, Minnesota: $156 million → education, social
- ♥ Wal-Mart Foundation, Bentonville, Arkansas: $272 million → community[7]

Companies are channeling a growing share of their donations outside the United States. According to the Chronicle of Philanthropy survey of giving by the largest U.S. businesses, in 2007 41 companies surveyed gave $2.5 billion in cash and products abroad compared with $2 billion in the previous year. This trend of international giving is expected to increase, particularly in emerging markets.[8]

In addition to giving money, corporations also often donate business strategy expertise and intellectual capital. For example, Deloitte & Touche employees volunteered to sort clothes for the Catholic Charities of Dallas thrift store event. They also improved the sales' system by implementing merchandising techniques, resulting in a 20% increase in the store's profit. Another new trend is corporations matching donations given by employees to approved organizations. This doubles the impact of their employee dollar donations and significantly helps nonprofit organizations.

Social enterprise is another growing trend. Some corporations encourage employee volunteerism in the community and promote action. There are wonderful examples of this in the corporate snapshot segment of this book. Two quick examples of corporate giving in action are:

- ♥ **Jazzercise International, Founded by Judi Sheppard Missett** in 1969, actively encourages its 7,200 energetic instructors and approximately 500,000 fit customers to give back to their communities in a myriad of ways. Through Employee Volunteer Programs, Judi offers her staff paid time off for charity work and community service. In addition, their franchisees host local/ regional Jazzercise benefit classes for charities of their choice. Together, they have raised over $26 million for various charitable organizations including the American Cancer Society, American Lung Association, and the American Heart Association. One example of "jazzercisers" stretching themselves to help others: their frequent local food drives for Stan Curtis' *USA Harvest* which feeds 2 million hungry people every day.

♥ **John and Peter Coors**, part of the heads-up Coors family which has two foundations (Castle Rock Foundation and Adolph Coors Foundation), also have hearts for Africa. They started the Circle of Light Foundation in 2002, which has helped bring electricity to more than 8,000 households in rural areas of the continent, donating more than $3 million to this glowing cause.

Community Giving ≈ Another growing trend across the country is giving as a group. Estimated giving by the nation's 707 community foundations rose to a record $3.6 billion in 2006. According to the Foundation Center, gifts received by these foundations hit a record level of $5.6 billion in 2005—up 45% from the previous year. Community foundations are attractive options for donors who want to avoid the expense and time commitment associated with maintaining a private foundation.

Global Giving ≈ Americans take care of people in need, both in our country and abroad. From a global perspective, in 2006 U.S. citizens privately sent more than $95.2 billion to aid people in developing countries, according to the Hudson Institute. This staggering amount is in addition to the $27.6 billion given by the U.S. government in foreign aid and private lending, and investing assistance of $69.2 billion.[9] In addition to the benevolence of individuals and our government, the United States pays 22% of the United Nations' budget.

A 2007 study conducted by psychologists found that people are happier when they spend money on others—such as giving to charity—than when they spend money on themselves. If that is true, happiness must abound in the hearts of many Americans!

The Giving of Volunteers

While money talks, it's the volunteers who make nonprofit organizations successful. Volunteers give above and beyond their responsibilities to work, family, and friends and do it willingly and compassionately. And the trend of those who say they volunteer is growing. Did you know that in 2007, 61 millions Americans provided more 8 billion hours of service valued at more than $157 billion, according to the Points of Light Institute?

USA Freedom Corps was established in 2002 and operates the www. volunteer.gov website, partnering with most of the major volunteer organizations. A few fast facts from USA Freedom Corps: the number of AmeriCorps volunteers has grown by 50% since 2002 to 75,000 young members each year, while Senior Corps has more than 500,000 volunteers annually. Over 1 million students volunteer each year through Learn and Serve America. Peace Corps has reached a 30-year high of more than 8,000 volunteers serving 74 countries. VolunteerMatch networks their 1.6 million members with more than 50,000 nonprofit organizations in need of a hand. The search-friendly database of USAFC includes more than 4 million volunteer opportunities from organizations across the country, organized geographically by ZIP code.

Teach for America applications have reached a new high—25,000 of the very brightest college graduates seek to serve two-year stints teaching in the inner cities of America. A 2001 study found that 63% of all college-age Americans have volunteered at a local school, hospital, or neighborhood center, served as tutors, or raised funds locally.[10]

And what about those volunteering abroad? Based on data from Independent Sector (independentsector.org), American volunteers contributed at least $2.76 billion worth of time to international programs in 2005.[11]

Charities in the United States

The number of 501(C)(3) U.S. charities has risen to well over 1 million, up from 600,000 in 1996. Some scholars say there might be as many as 300,000 additional charities that have not registered with the Internal Revenue Service, and those numbers do not reflect the estimated 300,000 to 400,000 religious congregations that are not required to register.[12]

What Makes a Passionary?

'Passionaries' is a word coined and trademarked to replace a term harder to understand: 'social entrepreneurs.' Passionaries see a social problem and envision a solution. In the profiles of this book, you will see creative ideas for tackling problems of homelessness, hunger, slavery, poverty, disease, and imprisonment. Passionaries are problem-solvers and real-life heroes, and the solutions they find pave the pathway for others to follow.

The "Power of One" represents the passionary with vision, determination, perseverance, and focused energy. Real social change comes from the "Power of One" + the nonprofit's volunteers and donors. Fundamental change in social problems almost never comes through government laws and mandates, but from people-power: person-to-person and nonprofit-to-human actions.

Ripples happen when a single drop hits the surface of still water; one ripple begets even more. Someone is touched, moved, or inspired by a passionary or a nonprofit organization; in turn that person "gives forward," creating more ripples. This forward motion of passing along goodness perpetuates into infinity as the ripples multiply, often unseen and unknown.

Americans are blessed with a tradition of giving that goes back to our forefathers who concluded the Declaration of Independence with these words: "...with a firm reliance on the protection of Divine Providence, we mutually pledge to each other our lives, our fortunes, and our sacred honor." Since then, God has smiled on do-gooders and good deeds, with true change happening and rippling over the land.

How Can I Make a Difference?

If you could change the world, what would you do? Whether you want to start, help build, or join in philanthropic actions, the secret to making a difference is as easy as ABC: Any Body Can → *with passion!*

P Pick your passion, ignite your heart—and read every profile in this book.

A Analyze possibilities and potentials of nonprofit organizations and learn from them.

S Study the purpose-driven methods of successful passionaries.

S Share your plan, strategize, and inspire others.

I Implement your plan: start doing something.

O Organize: every effort needs good organization and accountability.

N Network your vision, share possibilities, and create teams to fund raise.

Here's a hint to finding your passions: The easiest, quickest, and *most fun* way to do this is to join established groups that are making a difference together. Best bets:

- ♥ A local service group, i.e. Kiwanis, Rotary, Lions, or Optimists. A list of service groups can be found in the appendix of this book.

- ♥ Ask a local faith-based organization putting their faith into action.

- ♥ Look for a community foundation in your area—there are more than 700 nationally—and join it. There is usually a fee that is collectively given to charity. You will learn and work together, meet interesting seekers with giving hearts, and invest together in the lives of others. The largest community foundation in the country is the Tulsa Community Foundation with $900 million in assets—way to go, community foundations![13]

Although the media basically ignores the phenomenon, millions of Americans are actively turning their compassion into action and leaving a legacy of benevolence. Somewhere along the way, "do-gooder" became a negative term in some minds, but not in many hearts throughout this country. The world depends on these giving individuals, who often serve God by serving others. They are ordinary people doing extraordinary things together. In many ways, passionaries, volunteers, and donors represent the true spirit and heart of America the Beautiful. You, too, can make a difference in the world. Put your passion into action: Join, build, or start an effort ... just do something!

"I am only one, but I am one. I can't do everything, but I can do something. The something I ought to do, I can do. And by the grace of God, I will." —Edward Everett Hale

Foreword

Dr. Chuck Colson, Prison Fellowship

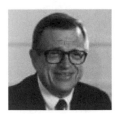 *Chuck Colson is a Watergate felon-turned prison evangelist, columnist, radio commentator, and founder and CEO of Prison Fellowship which currently offers services to the millions of incarcerated people and their families. He is the author of more than 20 books, including the international bestsellers "Born Again" and "How Now Shall We Live."*

Throughout His earthly ministry, Jesus showed a special concern for society's outcasts: the prostitute and the prisoner, the poor and the sick, the thirsty child and the victim of crime. These people mattered to Jesus. Do they matter as much to us?

I was once in the congregation of a Florida church when the pastor made a startling confession. "My message today is on the parable of the Good Samaritan," he announced. "Let me start with an illustration. Do you remember last year when the Browns came forward to join the church?" Everyone nodded. The Browns were an attractive, middle-class family. The pastor went on: "Well, that same morning a young man came forward. He gave his life to Christ that day."

Surprised murmurs rippled through the sanctuary. No one remembered the young man. The pastor went on: "Well, after that day we worked with the Browns, got them involved in the church, signed them onto committees. But the young man ... well, we could tell he needed help. We gave him counseling, but then lost track of him—that is, until yesterday." The pastor held up a newspaper. "He was charged with killing an elderly woman."

A hush fell over the congregation as the pastor continued: "I never followed up on that young man. And now I realize that I am the priest in the story of the Good Samaritan—the man who saw someone in trouble and crossed to the other side of the road. I am a hypocrite."

How easy it is for Christians to adopt the world's standards, judging people by how rich and powerful they are! But the church is true to its calling only when we radically reverse the values of the outside world.

The Passionaries in this chapter are doing just that. They rescue Asian children trafficked into sexual slavery, and offer blankets to homeless men shivering on American streets. They offer mentally challenged athletes a chance to compete, and comfort the terrorist's victims. They rescue children trafficked into sexual slavery, offer food to the desperately hungry, jobs and hope to the homeless sidelined on American Streets, hope and possibilities to those in prison and their families surviving at home, and fight for the future of our children both in our country and around the world.

While these "passionaries for humanity" are not necessarily Christian or faith-based stories, each of these remarkable individuals do follow in the footsteps of Christ, caring for those He called "the least of these."

Are you and I willing to do the same?

−Dr. Chuck Colson

CELEBRATING PASSIONARIES
WORKING AROUND THE WORLD

"Be the change you wish
to see in the world."
—Mahatma Gandhi

"Spread love everywhere you go.
Be the living expression of God's kindness."
—Mother Teresa

"If you don't know what your passion is,
realize that one reason
for your existence
on earth is to find it."
—Oprah Winfrey

"Even the turtle doesn't get ahead
unless he sticks his neck out."
—Dr. Robert A. Schuller

Kenneth Behring

Wheelchair Foundation

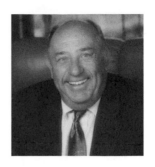

The Road to Purpose

Ken Behring discovered the true purpose of his life long after *Forbes Magazine* listed him as one of the 500 wealthiest men in America. It happened after his children all had children of their own, after he had built cities and owned a professional football team. It happened after he realized that material success couldn't bring him the fulfillment he so desperately desired.

Ken Behring was born dirt poor in Monroe, Wisconsin, during the Depression—a period of his life he calls the "more" phase. Those years were focused on meeting basic needs. His only clothes were a pair of overalls. His great pleasures were simple things like the opportunity to enjoy hot water or indoor plumbing. He joined his high school football team partly because it would give him an opportunity to take his first hot shower.

Ken's willingness to work hard to make his dreams come true was evident even at age six, when he began catching night crawlers and selling them for a nickel a can. He mowed lawns and caddied at the local golf course. When he had saved enough to purchase a bicycle, his young career moved into high gear. His new mobility allowed him to get a paper route, which in turn helped him recognize an early strategy for success: setting up newspaper sales outside a popular local drugstore, where he learned the importance of the old adage, "location, location, location."

In high school, Ken worked hard at studies, football, and work. He discovered that he loved people and enjoyed selling things—and he was good at it. With raw ambition and hard work, his bicycle was replaced by a car. Soon he started buying and selling cars. Eventually he talked the Chevy dealer into selling him the 27 cheapest used cars on the lot for $900—and Ken started his own used car lot, which he called Behring Motors.

Problems that might stump normal people became exciting challenges to Ken. When a massive snowstorm paralyzed Monroe, he turned the business setback into an opportunity, trading a truck and a car for a Jeep with a plow and clearing driveways and parking lots all over town. Within three years of starting Behring Lincoln-Mercury, 27-year-old Ken—the consummate people-lover and hard-working salesman—was making $50,000 a year and had $1 million in assets.

Ken calls the next phase of his life "better" when he focused his drive on attaining a higher quality lifestyle. Ken sold his car dealership and moved to Florida with his wife, Pat, and children. With great vision, an innovative style, and a high tolerance for risk, he challenged the world of real estate by starting Behring Construction. His real estate developments were wildly successful, and Ken parlayed them into major building developments in Seattle and a large community near San Francisco called Blackhawk.

Ken labels the third phase of his success as "different," as he shot for the "Lifestyles of the Rich and Famous." He assembled the world's largest classic car collection, bought a National Football League team (the Seattle Seahawks), and acquired his own private jet—a DC-9. But no matter how much more, better, and different things he accumulated, Ken still had an empty feeling in his heart. "No one had ever discussed or defined purpose for me, but I knew instinctively something was missing," he said.

"The real legacy I hope to leave is to get more people helping other people..."

In 2000, at the age of 72, Ken agreed to allow his private jet to be used to deliver wheelchairs to disabled people in Vietnam—and he agreed to go along on the trip. As he lifted a six-year-old Vietnamese girl off a pile of rags in the corner of her home and placed her in a wheelchair, Ken discovered what he had been searching for his whole life: purpose. Little Bui Thi Huyen's radiant smile of thanks changed the course of his life. Ken realized that a refurbished wheelchair meant this little girl could now go to school and create a future for herself.

As Ken and his friends delivered the other wheelchairs, they met disabled people who had come from far and wide on skateboards, in handcarts, crawling on their stomachs, or in the arms of family and friends. One boy, who had lost the use of his legs, scooted from place to place on a wooden plank. Ken recalled, "I got completely sold when this one Vietnamese lady came over and through the interpreter said, 'I really wanted to die, but now I don't want to.' I saw that mobility could make a difference between someone wanting to live and wanting to die."

All his life, Ken never wanted to get into projects unless he could make them big and successful. After his trip to Vietnam—and a subsequent trip to Guatemala—Ken established the Wheelchair Foundation, the most significant venture of his life. Initially funding it with $15 million, Ken challenged people to give $75 to sponsor a wheelchair and promised that his foundation would deliver it to someone in need. Through the fall of 2007, more than 625,000 wheelchairs have been distributed worldwide.

A multitude of partnerships with non-governmental organizations, foundations, service groups, corporations, and schools have helped spur the growth of the Wheelchair Foundation and kept costs down. Their 2001 partnership with Rotary Clubs International enabled them to reduce the cost of delivering 240 wheelchairs from $36,000 to $18,000. Working with Robert and Donna Schuller and friends from the Crystal Cathedral in Garden Grove, California, Ken made deliveries to Zambia, and his appearances on "The Hour of Power" television show raised donations for thousands of wheelchairs. The humanitarian arm of The Church of Jesus Christ of Latter-day Saints sponsors the delivery of tens of thousands of wheelchairs worldwide each year.

Deng Pufang (the son of China's late president, Deng Xiaoping) works ardently as a partner of the Wheelchair Foundation. In 1968, during the Cultural Revolution, Pufang's back was broken when he was pushed off a balcony. Confined to a wheelchair since that day, Pufang started the China Disabled Person's Federation (CDPF), which now has a chapter in every major city in China. "We have 35 million people in China who are disabled," said Ken, who is the only non-Chinese on that organization's board. "That gives you an idea of how big the scope of disability and need in China really is." Ken's groups make four trips a year to China, working with the CDPF to deliver where the need is greatest.

On one trip to Zimbabwe, Ken met a man who had crawled 12 miles on his elbows to get to the distribution center. Once seated in a wheelchair, he started pushing himself around and around. After about an hour in the chair, he pulled himself out and sat on the ground. Through an interpreter, Ken asked him, "Why did you get out of the wheelchair?" The man answered, "I've had my turn." Shocked, Ken responded, "This is your wheelchair." When the man explained that he had no money, Ken told him it was a gift, and the man was overjoyed and thankful. A year later, when the group went back to the same area of Zimbabwe, the man was there in his wheelchair, surrounded by children. "I came back 12 miles," he said, "because I want to show you that the wheelchair is just like new and my children want to thank you for what you have done for me."

Ken is still active in his for-profit businesses. Working alongside his sons, partners, and friends, he is making a significant impact on the world. He has achieved the pinnacle of business success and, by any standard, achieved the American dream through an insatiable work ethic and entrepreneurial spirit. He said candidly, "I like to make a lot of money and I like to spend a lot of money and I like to give a lot of money. I am still very big in the business world. The more you make, the more you can give, the more you can spend."

Ken learned that even late in life a person can re-chart life's course for significance and purpose. He has participated in hundreds of wheelchair distributions and seen many lives transformed by a simple gift of independence and mobility. The purposeful redirection of his life has altered the course of hundreds of thousands of other lives—not just immobile people but also the people caring for them. "We estimate that each wheelchair delivered improves the quality of at least 10 lives: parents, siblings, friends and caregivers," Ken said.

Every time Ken delivers a wheelchair, he follows the same routine: seating the person in the wheelchair, offering his hand, smiling expansively, and expressing the love of the people of the United States. "The real legacy I hope to leave is to get more people helping other people, so that after I'm gone, the work I've done will continue to multiply," Ken said. His life has gone from "more" to "better" to "different." Ken Behring has discovered joy, and the legacy of his purpose ripples around the world.

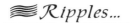

Justin Gonsalves, Boy Scout

Justin Gonsalves, a 17-year-old Boy Scout from Union City, California, loved attending Oakland A's baseball games so he could watch the inspiring play of Miguel Tejada, a shortstop known for his grand slam homeruns. During one of those games, Justin saw video footage of team members distributing wheelchairs in the Dominican Republic with the Wheelchair Foundation. Justin immediately decided to do something for the physically disabled as his Eagle Scout project.

After meeting with his troop leader, Justin planned a pancake breakfast fundraiser and a direct mail campaign. One of the key requirements for his project was to complete a minimum of 100 hours of community service. He pulled together a team and logged more than 130 hours of service, while raising $8,328.49 for the Wheelchair Foundation.

"It feels good to be a Boy Scout and help disabled people like this," Justin said. His donation enabled the Wheelchair Foundation to deliver 111 wheelchairs to physically disabled people in Mexico. Justin participated in the distribution, changing many lives—including his own.

Rotary International

Ken Behring is a member of the Rotary Club of Foster City, California, and knows firsthand the power of this service group to change the world. As a Wheelchair Foundation partner that caught Ken's vision early in 2001, Rotary Clubs and individual Rotarians have sponsored the delivery of more than 90,000 wheelchairs to 85 countries around the world. Rotarians from every state in the U.S.A. and every province in Canada have participated in the mission of getting wheelchairs to people in need of mobility.

Rotarians are an organization of 1.2 million business and professional leaders worldwide. They provide humanitarian service, encourage high ethical standards in their work, and help build goodwill and peace in the world. There are about 31,000 Rotary Clubs in more than 160 countries that live their motto: "Service above self."

Over the past 20 years, Rotarians have contributed more than $500 million toward the worldwide eradication of polio and coordinated National Immunization Days in India that have vaccinated up to 100 million people in a single day. Rotary Club leaders caught the vision of teaming up with the Wheelchair Foundation to deliver mobility to victims of polio who could not be helped by the vaccine. As many as 100,000 wheelchairs have been delivered to polio victims worldwide as a result.

One of the best reasons to be a member of a Rotary Club in North America is the heartwarming stories of friendship and gratitude brought back by members who have traveled abroad to participate in hands-on humanitarian service projects. On these missions of peace, they face the human reality that disease, advanced age, accidents, and land mines are the primary causes of physical disability worldwide. The Wheelchair Foundation works hand-in-hand with dedicated Rotarians worldwide to provide mobility for people in need.

Robert A. Schuller's Crystal Cathedral Church

With a dream as expansive as China, Pastor Robert A. Schuller and the members of his Crystal Cathedral have launched Silver Tiger, a mammoth vision of reaching out to 25 million residents of China's Gansu province. Gansu lies in northwestern China, extending from the north on the Mongolian border to the geographic center of China on the south. The 2,000-year-old Silk Road—the main trading route between China and Europe—passes through this area.

Inspired in part by their relationship with Ken Behring who has appeared on their Sunday morning *Hour of Power* television show, the dream of this Chinese mission has been percolating for a few years. The vision involves partnering with various nonprofit organizations to bring health, education, support, and hope to the Chinese mainland—primarily in Gansu province—through a six-pronged outreach:

♥ Working with the Wheelchair Foundation and the China Federation for Disabled Persons (CFDP), they will turn the spotlight on helping people with broken bodies by providing 8,000 wheelchairs.

- ♥ In partnership with the Dandelion Middle School, the Crystal Cathedral will provide education to the children of migrant workers.

- ♥ Alongside the Beijing International Committee for Chinese Orphans and a training program for Chinese foster parents, Crystal Cathedral supporters will provide physiotherapy and occupational therapy training for Chinese foster parents and social workers caring for handicapped children.

- ♥ Silver Tiger supporters will give scholarships and loans encouraging excellence in education, primarily helping exceptional middle school students continue their high school education when their compulsory education ends after the ninth grade.

- ♥ With Light Up the World Foundation, the Schullers' outreach includes promoting renewable energy and solar lighting technologies to bring affordable, safe, healthy, efficient, and environmentally responsible illumination to people in rural China.

- ♥ Together with the China Association for International Friendly Contact, they will focus on building water storage wells to provide safe drinking water for families in desperate need.

After arriving in Beijing in June 2001, David and Joy Rathbun began helping Dr. Schuller arrange meetings and publish books in China and set up a Chinese website. David and Joy, as a husband-and-wife team, have been working on a part-time basis for the Crystal Cathedral Ministries in China. They set up a one room office for the California-based Dr. Robert Schuller Institute for Possibility Thinking, Inc. Joy is an architect and designer, and David is a television journalist and writer.

The Schullers—along with the members and supporters of the Crystal Cathedral, David and Joy Rathbun, and a host of nonprofit organizations—will reach out in love and share positive possibility-thinking solutions to help the Chinese people. As they activate the dream and mobilize their members, we'll all watch the miracles multiply, rippling over Gansu province!

In 2000, Ken Behring founded the Wheelchair Foundation with a goal of delivering mobility to disabled people around the world, bringing hope, dignity, and freedom to the estimated 100 million people suffering from immobility. Through the fall of 2007, they have delivered more than 625,000 wheelchairs to countries in Africa, South America, the Middle East, and Asia, as well as to special places in the United States like the Walter Reed Army Medical Center in Washington, D.C. They distribute through an established network of organizations that are certified to import humanitarian aid duty-free and have established distribution channels in place. Behring's book, *The Road to Purpose*, is an inspirational roadmap to success in life.

To keep good works rolling forward to people in need, contact:

Wheelchair Foundation World Headquarters

3820 Blackhawk Road

Danville, California 94506, USA

Phone: (877) 378-3839 Toll Free — North America

Fax: (925) 791-2346

E-mail: info@wheelchairfoundation.org

Website: www.wheelchairfoundation.org

"Life is a blank check:
what it's worth depends
on how you fill it out."
—Proverb

Gary Haugen

International Justice Mission

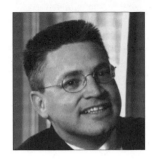

A Light Burning Brightly

Few people could have grown up farther from the realities of suffering and oppression in our world than Gary Haugen.

"I was raised in a wonderfully happy home, with a loving family, in an affluent suburb in Northern California," Gary said. "I knew little about the needs of the world. I knew even less about what those needs had to do with me, or how I could make a difference."

But that was about to change. Gary Haugen's adventures transformed his innocent youth into a deep passion to change the world for the oppressed.

At a young age, Gary was inspired by stories about two heroes who rose up against social injustice: President Abraham Lincoln, for his courageous stand to free American slaves, and Martin Luther King Jr., for his brave struggle against the brutality of segregation. "The drama of a single human being making such a difference in a world full of suffering and injustice captured my imagination," Gary said. "I was very earnest and very devout in my Christian faith and had this notion in my mind that there was just something that was found in places of suffering. I wanted to explore that. I felt personally convicted by Isaiah 1:17, which commands us to 'seek justice, encourage the oppressed, defend the cause of the fatherless [and] plead the case of the widow.'"

As a college student, Gary had met a man named Benigno "Ninoy" Aquino, who later was murdered when he returned to the Philippines to challenge the dictator Ferdinand Marcos. Aquino was brutally shot as he stepped off the plane. "Ever since [his death]," Gary said, "I've had an interest in human rights abuses in the Philippines."

After graduating from Harvard University in 1985, Haugen went to South Africa, where he spent a year with the National Initiative for Reconciliation. Working with Bishop Desmond Tutu and other church leaders, he witnessed firsthand the injustice and abuse of apartheid.

He saw people whipped and beaten by police, thrown into prison and tortured. "But in the midst of all that," Haugen recalled, "I got to see extremely brave and courageous people trying to do the right thing. They lived with a supreme lack of fear—and I wondered if I could live like that."

When Haugen returned to the United States, he entered the University of Chicago Law School because he saw law as the best avenue to create change. While in law school, Gary's work for the Lawyer's Committee for Human Rights took him to the Philippines where he led investigations into police abuse and military killings. That led to a position in the Civil Rights Division at the U.S. Department of Justice, where he investigated cases of police misconduct.

In 1994, Haugen was selected by the United Nations to head their investigation into the Rwandan genocide, during which 800,000 people from the Tutsi tribe had been hacked to death in just eight weeks by mobs of Hutu tribal people wielding machetes and farm implements. He walked through one mass gravesite after another, gathering evidence he hoped would indict the war criminals behind the massacre. His last stop was the lakeside village of Kibuye.

Haugen stood in Kibuye's spacious stone cathedral and listened to a harrowing account of what had taken place there: After the suspicious death of Rwanda's Hutu president earlier in the year, the provincial governor and mayor had ordered many of the local Tutsis into the cathedral to "keep them safe" from the chaos that was erupting in the area. When the Tutsis had gathered in the cathedral, Hutu radicals—including police officers—hacked through hundreds of men, women, and children. They attacked with machetes, spears, metal rods, and wooden clubs with nails sticking out. After slaughtering everyone in the cathedral, the mob made its way to the local stadium, where thousands of frightened, helpless Tutsis had taken refuge. The massacre at the stadium took so long that the killers decided to close off the stadium overnight so they could get a good night's rest before coming back to finish the job.

"Most of us are yearning for meaning and significance in our existence, but we figure, 'What difference could I make?' The answer is straightforward: If you want your light to burn brightly, take it into the darkness."

Gary knew that God hated injustice, but experiencing the gruesome nature of this injustice at point-blank range helped him understand the intensity of God's indignation.

When he returned to the United States, Gary set up meetings with friends and associates around Washington, D.C., who shared his Christian faith and desire to do something about the injustices they also had seen throughout the world. A 1996 survey of 40,000 overseas relief, development, and mission workers revealed that nearly 100% had seen abuses of power in their communities, but were powerless to stop it.

Those meetings led Gary to the greatest adventure of his life: founding International Justice Mission (IJM) in April 1997. IJM seeks to protect people from violent forces of injustice by securing rescue and restoration for victims and ensuring that public justice systems work for the poor. To this end, IJM lawyers, investigators, and aftercare professionals work with local governments to rescue victims, prosecute perpetrators, and strengthen public justice systems in communities.

"The last generation of human rights efforts focused on establishing international norms of acceptable behavior and getting many countries to change their laws in order to conform to those standards," Gary said. "Now there is a need for a vast army of people of good will who will do the hands-on work of making sure the actual victims of abuse get all of the benefits of the changes in the law over the past generation," he said.

It's been more than 10 years since Gary launched International Justice Mission, which now operates 14 offices in Asia, Africa, and Latin America. IJM takes on cases of slavery, sex trafficking, sexual abuse, illegal property seizure, illegal detention, and citizenship documentation. The group employs more than 200 people, but thousands of others have volunteered in one way or another, donating their time at headquarters in Washington, D.C., serving overseas, or supporting IJM through financial gifts or prayer.

"Most of us are yearning for meaning and significance in our existence, but we figure, 'What difference could I make?' The answer is straightforward: If you want your light to burn brightly, take it into the darkness," Gary said. "Think about it: If a great auditorium were fully lit, someone could light a match and almost no one would notice. But if that great room was thrown into pitch darkness and you were the one who lit a single match, no one in the auditorium would miss the miracle."

"We don't always know in advance precisely how we can make a difference, but we can work to make sure that doing nothing is *not* an option," he added. "We have tremendous capacities to render justice in the world if we just won't be overwhelmed. We simply need to step up to the point of need and render what we have."

Victories from IJM . . . Manna and Nagaraj

Manna lived with her brother and was beaten by him on several occasions. When she was 14, she decided running away was her best option. The clutter and scuffle of the train station frightened her, however, and Manna was grateful when a young woman offered to help. She listened to Manna and won her trust, promising to get her a job selling fabric. She then led Manna to a place where she could rest for the night, and even slept beside her. But when Manna woke the next morning, the woman who had helped her was gone. Another woman warned her that her life was no longer her own. Instead of selling fabric, she would have to work as a prostitute.

Manna refused her first three customers, but the brothel owner punched and beat her until she gave in to the men who had come to rape her. She tried to run away and even begged the men who raped her to rescue her or call the police.

The nightmare continued for two years until another girl who had been rescued by IJM led investigators back to the brothel to rescue more girls hidden in a soundproof dungeon. Manna was one of four girls rescued from that dark place. She now lives free in an aftercare home that provides love, safety, and the schooling she needs to become a social worker. IJM helped build a case against the brothel keepers, who were both convicted and sentenced to five years' rigorous imprisonment.

With a smile that brightens the room like sunlight, Manna said, "I came to prison, but I am not alone. God took me from that place to here. I am requesting that, like IJM saved me, they will save even more. What is impossible for men is possible for God."

For **Nagaraj**, the hope of freedom was stronger than the threats and abuses he and others endured while working in the brick factory. The worst part, he said, was seeing his children there, getting sick from excessive work in the searing heat, knowing they could never go to school and would grow up to become someone else's property. Nagaraj himself had been a slave since the age of 12. Their owner was a particularly brutal man who was feared in the community. No one dared to stand against him.

When IJM investigators and local authorities led a dramatic raid, 78 slaves were brought out of the kiln and given official release papers. A total of 138 people are now free men, women, and children. The owner was arrested to face criminal charges. IJM agents continued to monitor his case. IJM-supported social workers assisted the former slaves, ensuring they had the opportunities and resources they needed to establish free lives.

Many of the men freed from the kiln formed the Dawn Association, to provide a financial safety net for the families of those who have come out of slavery. If a member is in financial need, he can request a business or personal loan at a reasonable rate so the family won't fall prey to the economic trap of bonded slavery. Nagaraj was unanimously elected president of the Dawn Association and now runs his own brick kiln.

Nagaraj holds a brick in his hands as he tells his story to several visitors. "This is a brick I made from my own brick kiln. This is much better than what I used to build when I was in bondage. This is a very high quality stone. It is a brick made with free hands."

IJM: Zach Hunter

When a Virginia 7th grader, Zach Hunter, first learned from his mother that millions of people around the world—including children—are slaves, he knew he had to do something. Historical figures like Dr. Martin Luther King Jr., Mother Teresa, and William Wilberforce were among his heroes. When he learned that many slaves IJM rescues are children, Gary Haugen joined the ranks of his heroes.

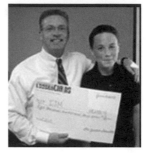

Remembering that many in America also used to face the oppression of slavery, Zach decided to empower and rally American students to fight slavery. "What I love about my generation is how expressive we are and how much we care about the world when we are confronted with issues of suffering and oppression," he said. "I'm excited about my generation. I'd like to see us become the peace, love and justice generation. But instead of doing it like the young people of the 60's and doing it without God—let's do it with God."

In an ABC News interview, Zach said, "There are actually 27 million slaves in the world. I was really surprised...and had all these emotions. But I knew that feeling bad was not enough—I had to do something." He shared facts: Human Rights Watch estimates that in South Asia alone as many as 15 million children are held in bonded slavery, whether working at brick kilns, chained to carpet looms, or working in rock quarries; many children are sold into slavery by family members to pay debts; and slaves are forced to work long, grueling days with little pay or hope, often beaten if they displease their owners. Then Zach talked about Gary Haugen's activities with IJM to stop slavery, concluding that modern-day slavery ought to be abolished and that people who get involved can make a difference.

Zach launched "Loose Change to Loosen Chains," challenging other kids to help emancipate slaves and create justice in the world. He encouraged students to collect loose change from their family and friends from late February through the first of April 2006. The students at Zach's school collected more than $8,500 and presented the money to Gary Haugen in person.

At age 15, Zach is a seasoned abolition advocate and now author of two books, *Generation: Change* and *Be the Change*, which have been translated into Spanish, Chinese, Czech and Braille. As he travels the country, he describes how William Wilberforce abolished the English slave trade in the early 1800s and how we can free slave children and their families today. This high-school crusader is speaking out about the slave problem as he continues to collect change that adds up.

For More Information

The U.S. Department of State declared in a 2006 Trafficking in Persons Report that "of the estimated 600,000 to 800,000 men, women, and children trafficked across international borders each year, approximately 80 percent are women and girls, and up to 50 percent are minors. The report also states that "the International Labor Organization—the United Nations agency charged with addressing labor standards, employment, and social protection issues—estimates there are 12.3 million people in forced labor, bonded labor, forced child labor, and sexual servitude at any given time; other estimates range from 4 million to 27 million." In April 1997, Gary Haugen founded International Justice Mission to combat these types of human rights abuses and ensure advocacy for the victims.

IJM works internationally through investigative casework and educational initiatives. To find out more, read Gary Haugen's book, *Good News about Injustice*, or visit their website, www.ijm.org.

Be a super-hero: fight for truth, justice and the IJM way. Contact:

International Justice Mission:

PO Box 58147

Washington, DC 20037-8147

Phone: (703) 465-5495

E-mail: contact@ijm.org

Website: www.ijm.org

Loose Change to Loosen Chains:

Start a club at your school by emailing Zach Hunter at loosechangetoloosenchains@gmail.com. Check out Zach's book: *Be the Change* or go to www.myspace.com/lc2lc

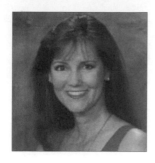

Nancy Rivard
Airline Ambassadors

Wings of Hope & 'Voluntourism'

In the early 1980s, Nancy Rivard was steadily climbing the corporate ladder at American Airlines. She'd been promoted from flight attendant to supervisor and was a budding executive. Hard work had earned her a Master's degree. Years of ambition and diligence were finally starting to pay dividends.

Then on a Christmas Eve, her father died unexpectedly of bladder cancer. "My dad was only 54-years-old. What if I died tomorrow?" thought 29-year-old Nancy. "I asked myself 'Do I feel right about what I'm doing?' And the truth was I didn't. What I·wanted was to know God and have a connection to something bigger."

Nancy made a bold decision to entirely start over. She gave away most of her possessions, relocated from California to Hawaii, and returned to her old job as a flight attendant. She took a substantial cut in pay, but gained the time and flexibility to search for spiritual answers. For seven years, Nancy's flight attendant status enabled her to take a trip every month, often to remote and unusual destinations—living with Hopi Indians and kibitzing with spiritual elders of a village high in the Andes Mountains of Peru. Witnessing firsthand the inequity between the haves and have-nots, a vision began to develop in Nancy's heart: using the travel industry to foster good will and understanding between diverse cultures. She saw children all over the world in desperate need of medicine, food, and other tangible goods that could be easily transported by plane.

"I had flown to Sri Lanka to visit little four-year-old Dinesha, a girl I had 'adopted' through Save the Children," Nancy said. "By the time I made it to her house with an armload of presents, I had 75 other children following me. It broke my heart that I did not have enough for all of them. They were so very grateful for anything, a pen, a ball...even a hug. I vowed to use my life to help these children, and children like them throughout the world."

At age 30, Nancy and her boyfriend were sitting on a beach in Hawaii when her boyfriend proposed. Her reaction surprised even her: "I remember pounding my hand on the sand and saying, 'I just can't marry you.' I realized my mission was to use my life somehow in a way to benefit humanity." Turning down the proposal, Nancy asked her fellow flight attendants for help. "They weren't in the least bit interested," she said. "So I thought, if I can't get anybody to go with me, I'll do it by myself. And I did."

At first, Nancy took a few days each month to put her flight attendant travels to good use. She visited refugees in Bosnia, handing out hundreds of tiny hotel products collected on layovers. Then she used one of her flights to help a little girl who needed heart surgery get from Guatemala to New York City. When her colleagues saw Rivard beaming with joy from her philanthropic travels, they began asking how they could help. Soon Nancy had a notebook full of names. All she had to do then was ask people on her travels what they needed most and match them up with an attendant flying in that area.

Nancy likes to call her trips "voluntourism," a combination of "volunteering" and "tourism."

In 1996, Nancy moved to Washington, D.C., with the intention of making congressional contacts and starting the nonprofit effort, which she named Airline Ambassadors International (AAI). With a lot of dedicated work, AAI grew into a network of hundreds of flight attendants and others traveling the world to deliver supplies, medicine, and food to nations in need, even uniting adoptive parents with their children.

Nancy likes to call her trips "voluntourism," a combination of "volunteering" and "tourism," resulting in unforgettable travel. On every AAI mission, she includes time for enjoying the destination as well as delivering school supplies, medicine, shoes, soccer balls, hygiene products, and needed incidentals. Her volunteers pay their own expenses, helping out at clinics, schools, or orphanages, as well as exploring local sites. These trips create memories for a lifetime—for both the recipients and the travelers.

By 2007, AAI had hand-delivered $50 million worth of donations to 51 countries and 15 U.S. cities. Since Nancy Rivard's first solo trips,

Airline Ambassadors has signed up more than 6,000 members and volunteers who, in addition to delivering donations, have escorted more than 1,000 children to adoptive homes and medical centers.

"What we have accomplished is incredible," said Nancy, who has been featured on several syndicated news shows. More than 100 national and international magazines and newspapers have covered stories of the amazing work being done by Nancy and AAI's traveling Samaritans. In April 2007, NBC Nightly News featured Airline Ambassadors as a prime example of a new trend in "volunteer vacations."

Today, half of Airline Ambassador's volunteers are airline personnel, but a growing number are students, health and business professionals, homemakers, and retirees. AAI gives ordinary people a unique opportunity to experience the joys of hands-on relief work for themselves.

Nancy took a leave of absence from the airline in 2002 to run the organization with virtually no paid staff. Because of its explosive growth, AAI continues to need administrative personnel and regular sources of funding. As of 2004, Nancy and AAI, amazingly, still had no major foundation support or corporate sponsors.

Remarkably, Airline Ambassadors delivers $35 in aid for every $1 donated. "The only reason we are able to do this is because so many people sacrifice so much, donating their expenses as well as their time. Last year, AAI volunteers spent $500,000 to $1 million of their own money to do humanitarian work. The generosity and passion of our members is stunning," Nancy said. "There is a growing public out there that wants to make a difference across borders. This is their opportunity to bridge world need with world resources."

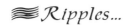

Children's Escort Program: Escorting Oliver

The responsibility of escorting a child in need was enough to make me a little nervous, especially when it was someone like Oliver, a 14-month-old boy with a heart condition. When I arrived in Honduras and saw Oliver and his family, I knew it would be ok. When his mother gave him to me, I was expecting tears and screams. But he looked up at me as though he knew I was taking him to make him better. Off to Chicago we flew, to take Oliver to "Healing the Children," an organization that arranges for desperately needed pediatric medical care. I had anticipated that being an escort would be rewarding, but I didn't realize the depth of my experience until I took Oliver back home to his grateful parents—as good as new! We all just cried and cried! His parents gave me a plaque that read, "Thank you, Rhonda, for helping our Oliver." It now hangs on my wall. Escorting children is a heartfelt experience you will never forget.

—Rhonda Bostock

Welcome to America, Semegne

Semegne looked so small and frightened. How in the world would I be able to reassure or comfort her? I didn't even speak her language. Semegne was an Ethiopian orphan who had traveled all the way from Addis Ababa to Newark, Pennsylvania, where I joined her for the last leg of the journey. Together, we flew to Charleston, South Carolina, to meet her adoptive family. With two hours before our flight, we got acquainted over frozen yogurt, snapping photos with my digital camera and showing her the images. Finally she gave me a big smile! Arriving in Charleston, Mom, Dad, and brother Jeremy were waiting. It was an incredibly moving moment, and there were few dry eyes around. Semegne's new family graciously invited me to share a meal with them before my return flight. On the drive to the airport, Jeremy explained to Semegne that they would soon be home. She tipped her face up to her new dad, and with a big smile said her first English word, "home," in a voice deeper and stronger than we expected. Yes, Semegne, you are finally home.

—Dawn Roe

Since its inception in 1996, Nancy Rivard's Airline Ambassadors (AAI) has hand delivered more than $50 million worth of medicine, medical supplies, school supplies, clothing, and food on missions to 15 U.S. cities and 44 countries around the world. More than 1,000 children have been escorted to new homes or to a destination where they received medical care not available in their home countries. More than 70,000 school children are involved in humanitarian activities, instilling compassion and encouraging creative thinking about solutions to the global issues that affect us all.

Because AAI operates on an annual budget of less than $180,000 per year, all mission participants pay their own expenses. Last year, volunteer members donated time and aid worth more than $500,000. More than 6,000 health professionals, business executives, housewives, teachers, students, and most of all the airline personnel, help children through AAI from all over the world.

Fly high! *Lift the hearts and hopes of others in need. Contact:*

Airlines Ambassadors International

418 California Avenue

PO Box 459

Moss Beach, California 94038

Phone: (866) ANGEL-86

E-mail: info@airlineamb.org

Website: www.airlineamb.org

"I wondered why somebody
didn't do something.
Then I realized: I am somebody."
—Anonymous

Chris Crane
Opportunity International

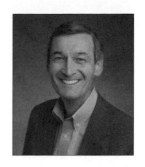

Passion to Help God's Beloved Poor

In the United States, we think an entrepreneur is someone who starts a business, usually with considerable initiative and risk. In our world, people *choose* to become entrepreneurs. If they fail, they do something else. If they succeed, they often become wealthy.

In the developing world, on the other hand, where three billion people live on less than $2 a day, being an entrepreneur is a matter of sheer *survival*, rather than choice. There, an entrepreneur faces a much different proposition. The alternative to succeeding in business—whether it is selling bananas at a stand, sewing clothes or making crafts—is losing a child to a perfectly curable illness, being forced to sell your children into slavery, or even watching your family starve.

Chris Crane is a very successful American-style entrepreneur who found his mission in life: helping entrepreneurs in the world's poorest countries succeed in business and raise themselves out of poverty. As a volunteer and supporter, Chris had experienced firsthand the power of giving micro-credit loans ($50 to 150) to the world's poor. His passion was ignited which led to his becoming the president of one of the world's largest micro-finance organizations. He was ready for a new challenge.

In 2002, Opportunity International asked Chris to lead the U.S.-based organization, one of the world's largest and fastest growing micro-finance organizations. Opportunity International helps poor entrepreneurs work their way out of poverty with $100 loans and business training. In 2007, more than 1.7 million poor entrepreneurs received $500 million. Ninety-eight percent of the loans were paid back, to be loaned again and again to millions of the poor in the coming years. Chris has helped leverage his business skills to get a big bang for his nonprofit's donors—to such an extent that for each dollar someone donates, the third-world poor receive $2.74.

Today Chris is president and CEO of Opportunity International. He doesn't accept a salary and pays his own travel expenses for the more than

150 days each year he spends on the road, fulfilling his commitment to the call to serve the poor.

The timing of his company's sale and the chance to join Opportunity International was "grace," Chris said. "When I first learned about Opportunity International, the entrepreneur and capitalist in me was just amazed that you could help poor entrepreneurs work their way out of poverty with so little investment."

God's grace has been evident in succeeding years as well. A tall, lanky man with an effervescent smile and seemingly boundless energy, Chris has led the organization to a 26% annual growth rate over the past five years.

Chris and Opportunity International are a powerful force in bringing a vision of transformation to impoverished women and men—"God's beloved poor," as he often refers to them. "It's absolutely thrilling. Our clients overseas are the most amazing, marvelous people. They do so much with so little money, and they work so hard because, for most of them, it's the only chance they'll ever have to work their way out of poverty."

"People work themselves out of poverty and do so with pride and a sense of empowerment."

Today, Opportunity International is helping more than eight million poor people in 28 countries of Africa, Asia, Eastern Europe, and Latin America. One million are loan clients who have received sometimes as little as $50 or $100 to start or expand a business so they can provide for their families and contribute to their communities. The principal lending methodology is a "Trust Group," about 20 to 30 entrepreneurs who guarantee each other's loans. Opportunity provides training, which runs the gamut from basic business practices, such as recordkeeping, to HIV/AIDS awareness education.

Micro-finance works where other international aid programs fail. "People work *themselves* out of poverty and do so with pride and a sense of empowerment," Chris explained. "Our clients feed and educate their children, grow their businesses, hire their neighbors and many become leaders in their communities, all of which contribute to helping break the chain of poverty."

During Chris' tenure, Opportunity International has expanded well beyond loans. "We realized that the poor needed access to the same kinds of financial services that we in the United States enjoy and take for granted, so we started building banks that exclusively serve the poor," Chris said. Since 2000, the organization has opened 17 institutions offering loans, savings accounts, and other financial services to people who never before had access to a bank.

"In most of the countries we operate, traditional banks serve only the wealthiest people. Their guards turn away the poor before they can even enter. At our bank, our guard smiles and welcomes them," Chris said. "If the clients cannot read, which is often the case, trained staff take them through the process of opening a savings account. Many times, people come in to make a very small deposit, such as $10, and then come back the next day to withdraw the money, just to make sure we will return their money. Once they know their money is safe, they'll come back and make larger deposits."

Those savings accounts help not just the entrepreneurs' families, but also the community at large and even the entire country. Money once kept in a coffee can buried in a hut—"dead capital"—can be put to work in the form of loans to other poor entrepreneurs who will employ people, produce products, and deliver needed services.

Insurance is another basic need that poor people in the developing world seldom have available. Opportunity International launched a program that offers credit and life insurance in Uganda, where life expectancy is less than 40 years of age. As people learned the value of insurance, the business began to grow, and now Opportunity International's Micro-Insurance Agency insures 3.5 million people in 10 Asian and African countries, helping establish a financial safety net for the poorest of the working poor.

"With average premiums of about $1.50 per month, we're making affordable credit and life insurance available to those most at risk," Chris explained. "We even created a policy that insures people who are HIV positive or AIDS infected. We've developed new products like crop insurance in Malawi that, with the support of the World Bank, is being expanded to more countries in Africa. And we're now working toward creating affordable health insurance for the poor."

In 2007, Chris' team took on another bold initiative, becoming one of the first micro-finance organizations to fund "schools for the poor." These schools are operated primarily by women who are former teachers, located in the poorest neighborhoods, close to the students' homes. "This is particularly important for providing an equal opportunity for girls to attend school, since parents tell us they feel safer with their girls closer to home," Chris explained.

Now Micro-schools of Opportunity™ are operating in more than 50 poor neighborhoods in Ghana, with plans for rapid expansion in Africa and Asia. Schools in the pilot program have a remarkable student/ teacher ratio of 30-to-1, compared with 70-to-1 in government schools. The result is that children in these schools have performed above average on standardized tests. New research indicates that schools for the poor outperform their government school counterparts in several African countries, India, and China.

"Education is a new frontier in micro-finance and we are pleased to be leading the way. It is the third leg of the stool, along with banks and insurance, to help the poor escape poverty and to transform their lives once and for all," Chris said.

Does Chris feel overwhelmed by the task of ending poverty in this world?

"We cannot be afraid," he said. "We are put on this earth to glorify God, and it is by taking on the seemingly insurmountable problems of our world that we demonstrate his power and grace. In the same way, our clients face God-sized challenges every day and they persevere, with his help."

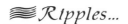

Small Loans Lead to Big School ≈ Dorothy Njobvu Kanjautso

After her husband's death from AIDS, Dorothy Njobvu Kanjautso's world was about to come apart. The 27-year-old mother found herself unable to provide for her three children. With what little money she had, Dorothy started a small nursery school—converting one of the two rooms in her tiny home into a classroom and hiring a teacher. But after a few months, the business began to decline. She was faced with being forced to beg to feed her children.

Instead, Dorothy discovered and joined an Opportunity International "Trust Group" in her village outside Lilongwe, the capital of Malawi, Africa. With a $70 loan from Opportunity International, she purchased play mats and games for the children. Her nursery school began to grow. With another loan, she expanded into a small elementary school for children who could not afford the travel or expense of attending a public school. Over four years, she built the school, grade-by-grade, child-by-child. She expanded to the sixth grade and hired seven teachers to serve more than 250 students. The 30-to-1 teacher-student ratio is far more favorable than the 70-to-1 ratio found in government schools.

With the business training she received in Trust Group meetings and her own initiative, Dorothy started two other businesses—an apartment building and a frozen treats stand near the school. She employs five other adults in those businesses—employees who can now afford to provide for their families thanks to Dorothy's entrepreneurial spirit and success.

Dorothy cares for the sick and orphaned, helping those who are HIV-positive and educating youth about AIDS and nutrition. She cares for her mother, fully supports three orphans, and provides free tuition at her school for five other AIDS orphans. She also encourages other women to start businesses in the community.

At home, the loans have improved both the nutrition and education of her children. Kelvin, 12, Natasha, 11, and Vanessa, 9, used to eat meat only once a month, but now they enjoy it weekly. Although she was recently diagnosed as HIV positive, she is investing the profits from her business so she can afford to educate her children all the way through college, which she hopes will give them the fighting chance to escape poverty.

"I dream for a future in the business," Dorothy said. "I want to have savings, but more than that I want to inspire courage in my children. I want my daughter to grow up to be a doctor, so she can help those in my country who are HIV-positive."

For More Information

Opportunity International is committed to solving global poverty. Serving more than 1.2 million poor entrepreneurs in 28 developing countries, Opportunity International is a pioneer in offering small business loans, savings, insurance, and training in basic business practices to women and men living in chronic poverty. Founded in 1971 as one of the first microcredit lenders, Opportunity International provides small loans—sometimes as little as $50—and other services that allow poor entrepreneurs to start or expand a business, develop a steady income, provide for their families and create jobs for their neighbors. Opportunity International is motivated by a call to serve the poor and maintains a network of offices across the globe, with United States offices in Oak Brook, Illinois and San Diego, California.

Don't miss this lifetime opportunity to use microcredits to make macro-changes. Call:

Opportunity International USA

2122 York Road

Oak Brook, Illinois 60523

Phone: (630) 242-4100 | Fax: (630) 645-1458

Website: www.opportunity.org

For a new and exciting way to give online—check out OptINnow at optinnow.org.

Haiti Calling

The following three stories are of people called to help the poor in the Third World country of Haiti. Just a mere 500 miles from the shores of the United States, the lure of need and love calls to the hearts of three magnificent Americans. This is but the tip of the iceberg; people from around the world are reaching out to Haiti, which cries out in need to helping hearts.

Susie Scott Krabacher
The Mercy and Sharing Foundation

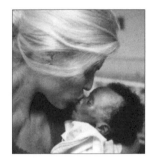

For the Love of Children in Poverty

Susie Scott Krabacher was having a rare smoke outside the government hospital in Port-au-Prince, Haiti, when a frail, bent woman approached her and tugged her arm.

"Come," the woman told her.

Susie followed. The woman led her to a narrow alley between two concrete buildings. In that alley lay a torn piece of cardboard on which lay a little girl, around four or five years old, who couldn't have weighed more than 20 pounds. She wore a dirty blue dress; faded plastic hair clips held her braided hair. She was curled in the fetal position, and her bone-thin legs twisted unnaturally.

Susie noticed the girl's dress was soiled and ripped around her pelvis area. She pulled back the torn cloth to reveal the girl's hipbone protruding through her skin. Countless parasites had infested the wound. Susie picked up the girl and turned to look for the old woman, but she was gone.

Holding the girl tightly, Susie hurried back to her hotel, where she held the girl, rocking and singing to her until a doctor came. The doctor visited often during the next several days. Finally, the girl was well enough to be transported to an orphanage Susie had started years ago in Port-au-Prince. They named the child Vicki.

When Susie and her husband, Joe, celebrated their anniversary a few months later, they gave each other what Susie remembers as the best anniversary present ever. They used the money they would have spent on gifts to have a skin graft taken from Vicki's back to cover her hip bone.

Vicki became a well-nourished child in the clean, secure, loving environment of the orphanage, but she also struggled with cerebral palsy, which often made her sick. Despite the medical care she was given, Vicki died. But unlike so many of Haiti's children, she died in dignity, surrounded by people who loved her.

Susie Scott Krabacher wasn't always the type to walk around Haiti's back alleys. She grew up in Alabama, where she was abused sexually, physically, and verbally by adult family members. But as a child, Susie experienced a moment of clarity one day. "I knew that someday I would do something significant, more significant than all these people who were hurting me could ever imagine," she said. "I promised God that I would fix it so no child ever suffered like I had again."

It would be a while, though, before those childhood dreams were realized. At the age of 15, Susie and her family moved to Utah, where she dropped out of school. Sixty-three days before she turned 16, she moved out of her parents' house. At the request of a photographer friend, Susie agreed to pose for a *Playboy* magazine test shoot. At 18, she was *Playboy's* May 1983 centerfold.

Susie dated a long string of men and relied on cocaine and scotch to get her through each day. After a failed marriage, she met and married attorney Joe Krabacher. Six years into the marriage, Suzie still struggled with low self-esteem and feeling she had little to offer her husband or anyone else. Then one night she flipped on the television and saw a boy in Mongolia who ate sewer rats to survive. "There on my couch in Aspen, in one brief, terrifying, unyielding, everlasting moment, everything changed," Susie said. "The Mongolian sewer boy and I had the same gash—the same hurting, hungry, screaming, lifelong wound. I wondered if he would be alive tomorrow. For the first time, I glimpsed a worse place to grow up than my mother's house in Alabama."

Determined to make a difference, Susie purchased a plane ticket to Mongolia. She ran into a man at church who had been to Haiti, a country

Susie and Joe had never heard of before. He was sure Mongolia's poverty would not compare to what he had witnessed in Haiti, and proved his point by showing Susie and Joe photo after heartbreaking photo of Haiti's desperate children. The next morning, Susie was on the phone, changing her Mongolia ticket to Haiti.

Susie arrived in Haiti in April 1994 with no plan, just a desire to help children. To better understand the demons Haiti's people were struggling against, Susie spent a night in Cite-Soleil, Haiti's poorest and most dangerous slum and home for 200,000 to 300,000 people, including many armed gang members.

She also visited the government hospital in Port-au-Prince, Haiti's capital city. As she walked through the Pediatric Unit, she found Ti-Judith, an emaciated baby wrapped in rags and lying in a rusted crib. Ants crawled in her dirty diaper, and her obviously ill mother leaned over the crib weeping. Susie cleaned the baby and found food for the mother. When she returned the next day, the baby's mother had died of AIDS. The next morning, Ti-Judith was also dead. Susie went to the morgue, where decaying corpses were piled around the room. After searching through stack after stack of bodies, Susie finally found Ti-Judith. She took the girl, bought her a clean dress, and buried her in the city cemetery. In Ti-Judith's coffin, Susie included a slip of paper that said: "In this world, you were loved." Since then, she's seen many other children die in the harsh conditions of Haiti and places the same note in the coffin of each child who dies in her care.

On that first trip to Haiti, Susie became convinced of the country's needs. With $12,000 left from a failed antiques business, she founded the Mercy and Sharing Foundation. As she established the fledgling organization, Susie drew strength from her faith and her fierce love for Haiti's children. As she learned the ropes of working in Haiti, she spent many hours reading the Bible and searching for direction. The foundation's first objective was to build a feeding center in Cite-Soleil. Despite setbacks including Susie being cheated out of funds, the feeding center (which became known as the Mercy Nutrition Center) soon opened. Eventually it began educating children too.

Today, more than 14 years later, Mercy and Sharing Foundation operates six schools and three orphanages, one of which serves only terminally ill children. An abandoned baby unit provides a place for impoverished mothers to safely leave their children, rather than abandoning them on the streets. They also feed thousands of people each month through nutrition programs in rural areas. A Mercy and Sharing community medical clinic is working to establish a screening program for cervical cancer, which Susie said is the biggest killer of Haiti's women.

Every dollar given to Mercy and Sharing goes directly to the programs in Haiti. Though Susie serves as the organization's president and CEO and dedicates most of her waking hours to Haiti's children, she has never received a salary. For Susie, seeing children loved, cared for, and given a chance for a better life is enough.

One of those children is a boy named Johnny. Susie saw him wandering near the government hospital. A nearby merchant told her his mother had died and he didn't know his father. He had been begging the merchants for food each day for two weeks. Susie took him to her hotel and gave him food and water. Now he calls one of the Mercy and Sharing orphanages home, and he's grown into a handsome, happy, and smart child.

Another child, David, was paralyzed when he arrived at Mercy and Sharing. The foundation provided a wheelchair for him, but one afternoon Susie heard one of the foundation board members laughing and shouting in the orphanage courtyard: "All right! That a boy! Come on, little man! You're doing it!" Susie saw David taking tentative steps with only the help of a walker.

Once, when Haiti was experiencing a period of even greater unrest than usual, a bounty was placed on Susie's head and friends tried to convince her to find someone else to do her work. Susie knew she would never find anyone else because of her self-written job description: "Must work impossibly long hours with little sleep. Must be willing to bury friends and children. Able to maneuver through coup d'etats and gang violence without losing supplies and getting shot at. Must have extraordinary personal radar to detect betrayal among friends and staff. Salary...oh, there is none."

Susie isn't overwhelmed by Haiti's darkness, though. In fact, she sees light there—tiny points of light in each child.

The Mercy and Sharing Foundation focuses its work on the island nation of Haiti, home to around 8 million people, including close to 6 million children. Haiti is generally accepted as the western hemisphere's poorest nation, where overpopulation and environmental degradation have led to what some view as hellish conditions. More than 70 percent of Haitians are unemployed. Those who do have jobs make an average of US $150 per year.

Mercy and Sharing cares for more than 3,000 children, orphans, and handicapped children through six schools, three orphanages, nutrition programs, and a medical clinic. The foundation believes not in charity, but in opportunity. They teach children and, in turn, the children learn and teach others. They feed children, and then teach the children to feed themselves and feed others. They educate children and teach trades to adolescents, empowering them to provide for themselves and their families. As the native Haitian staff members mentor, nurture, love, and respect the children, the children learn to love and respect others.

Mercy and Sharing welcomes people to donate their time, effort, and even finances. General volunteers and medical workers—like physicians, nurses, physical therapists, and dental hygienists—are needed to share their love and expertise with Haiti's youngest citizens. Every dollar donated to Mercy and Sharing goes directly to care for Haiti's children.

Be an angel ≈ give wings of love to Haitian children in desperate need of your compassion.

Learn more at www.haitichildren.com or (877) HAITI-KIDS, or contact Founder and CEO, Susie Scott Krabacher at: susie@haitichildren.com.

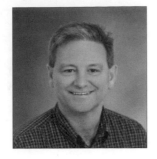

Scott Sabin
Floresta

Healing the Land and Its People

Standing on the street corner in the tiny California coastal town of Solana Beach, Scott Sabin could hear sirens blaring from blocks away and see smoke graying the distant horizon. "I was only seven or eight, but I remember standing there and watching those civil defense trucks roar down the street and out of town to fight the fires," Scott said. "I just felt this incredible pull to go with them and help those people—to put out the fires that were ruining their lives." That was the first glimpse of a heart for helping people in need that eventually would lead him to rebuild mountains.

Scott's desire to put out the proverbial fires in people's lives led him to the Navy after college, where he served as an officer for seven years. "Like many young people, I was on trajectory," Scott said. "Once I got out of the Navy, I went back to school to get my master's degree in international relations. I thought I was headed for the State Department to work as a diplomat." God had other plans. "Late into my program, I realized I needed either two years of classes or complete fluency in a foreign language." That was when Scott met Ken Souder, the executive director of an organization called Floresta, which worked in Third World countries to help the poor and reverse deforestation. Ken told Scott that if he wanted to become fluent in Spanish quickly, Guatemala was the place to do it.

"I couldn't quite see God's work in all of this at the time, but looking back on it, it's amazing how much He did to influence my heart," Scott recalled. He started asking around about Guatemala, and his roommate mentioned that his sister had traveled extensively and was giving a talk about her adventures. They went to hear her speak. "This woman was amazing," Scotts said. "She'd been everywhere, and she told incredible stories about her travels, including how she saw a dentist in rural China who had used a power drill to give her a root canal! I was hooked. It made me realize I really needed to stretch myself while I had the opportunity." Scott bought a ticket to Guatemala the next day, with no idea where he would go or how he would learn Spanish.

What he didn't know was that God would steal his heart in Guatemala.

While he was in the country, Scott ran into some young Presbyterian missionaries from Los Angeles. They told him about an amazing pastor named Solomon Hernandez, who lived in the hills outside Quiché. "Quiché was right in the heart of a civil war battle zone between the guerillas and the Guatemalan army," Scott explained. "But these kids were so deeply in awe of Solomon, I felt compelled to go up and meet him."

Scott traveled by bus for more than ten hours to reach Quiché, then hopped on a farm truck that was carrying bags of rice and about 30 other people into the mountains. Reaching the village of Uspantan, he stayed with Solomon for several days, looking at the work he was doing with orphans and the rural poor. "Solomon was a man who just loved life," Scott recalled. "He saw everything as a miracle, and he loved to laugh. And this had a huge, huge effect on me. This man was giving his life to others amidst poverty and violence and destruction—and he was joyful! At that moment, it was like my eyes were opened for the first time. I could see God's work through this man serving the people around him. He had nothing of worldly value, but loved life more than anyone I'd ever met."

"I just felt this incredible pull to go with them and help those people—to put out the fires that were ruining their lives."

Scott returned home a changed man, completed his degree and began looking for a role that would allow him to serve the poor. He approached Ken Souder at Floresta, which had only two employees and was working in one small area of the Dominican Republic, and offered to volunteer.

Floresta was founded in 1985 on the premise that poverty and environmental degradation go hand-in-hand. Deforestation is among the major causes of poverty and human suffering in places where people seek to stave off drought and famine by clearing forests or cutting down their own crop-bearing trees to sell as firewood or charcoal. Without trees, rainwater does not infiltrate the soil. Instead it runs off, eroding precious topsoil and stealing nutrients and water needed to irrigate crops. To make matters worse, the lack of forest cover decreases the amount of rainfall, resulting in much drier soil. And when rain finally does fall, flash flooding and mudslides often cause death and destruction. This drier climate and subsequent decrease in soil fertility make it difficult to farm, deepening the people's poverty and fueling the cycle all over again.

Through Scott's travels with Floresta, he repeatedly saw people forced to trade their future to survive for the present. "No amount of environmental education can change the actions of an individual desperate to survive," Scott said. "What all these people lack are alternatives, not education. And that's what we do at Floresta: give the poor viable options to shape successful futures for themselves and protect the environment." Scott's work and his belief in the potential of impoverished people to solve their own problems—when given the right opportunities—made a huge impact on Floresta. In 1995, Scott was hired to run the nonprofit.

As executive director, Scott was receiving repeated invitations from an Episcopal priest to work in Port Au Prince, Haiti. "As an organization, we had always thought we'd never go to Haiti," Scott said. "The culture is different; the language is different. At the time, it was literally a graveyard of good intentions gone awry. But this priest, Pere Albert, was insistent, and his spirit reminded me of my brother in Guatemala, Solomon Hernandez. So I convinced my country director to take me into Haiti to meet him."

Although they occupy the same island, Haiti and the Dominican Republic couldn't be farther apart. The countries are sharply divided. A border crossing requires multiple days of paperwork and government approvals. "We left from Santo Domingo for Port Au Prince and got held at the border for 36 hours," Scott recalled. "So by the time we arrived at the agreed location in Port Au Prince, no one was there to meet us. I knew his church was in the mountains in Cheridente, but this was Haiti! The level of poverty was just staggering, even by Third World standards. And the country was a dangerous place at the time, especially after dark." Using what little French they knew, Scott and his country director began asking people randomly if they knew Pere Albert, until they finally found a little girl who recognized the name. "I knew she knew him because when we said his name, her face lit up and she hopped right in the jeep," Scott said.

After several hours of searching, they finally found the little green church in Cheridente and met Pere Albert. He was another man truly after God's own heart, and he drew Scott and Floresta into Haiti almost immediately.

In Haiti, Scott was able right away to put all he had learned to work. He recognized that planting new trees in Haiti's mountains would reduce erosion levels, improve soil quality, and increase crop yields. It also would contribute to a cleaner, more plentiful water supply. He also knew that reversing the economic slide would reverse the environmental slide as well. So he set about teaching new farming skills, awarding micro loans to start small businesses, and planting trees—all with the help of the dedicated staff and volunteers of Floresta.

The small village of Kavanac, perched high in the southern mountains, was one of the first Haitian communities in which Floresta began working. Scott recalled an initial meeting with the villagers: "We had a community meeting with about 50 farmers. They were a really dejected group, and a couple of them had come up to me before the meeting asking for money. During the meeting, an older woman stood up and challenged me saying, 'UNICEF was here. They gave us food and left.' She went on to list two of three other agencies that had been involved in the area, with a similar outcome. 'How are you going to be any different?' I told her, 'First of all, we are not going to *give* you anything. Secondly we are not going to leave until you are ready to stand on your own two feet.'"

Years later, Scott visited Kavanac again, at a similar community meeting but this time attended by nearly 100 farmers. A woman stood and talked about her experience of Floresta. "She excitedly shared Floresta had given her village the confidence and knowledge to know that they were not helpless and that they could use their God-given talents to improve their own situation!" Scott said. "To me, that represented one of our most important accomplishments."

The people of Kavanac have improved their situation. With Floresta's help, they formed a credit cooperative which has made and collected hundreds of small business loans. They have planted thousands of trees, improved their crop yields, and learned to work together. As Floresta grows, it maintains the same goals and aspirations it held when Scott first came on board. "As a community begins to gain hope, they realize that they do have talents," he said. "They gain confidence, and the stars within the group emerge—people of tremendous talent who have lacked only opportunity and self-confidence. I think of my good friend Cheristone Bijou, truly one of the most remarkable people I have ever met. Despite the fact that he has only a third-grade education, Cheristone has gone from landless sharecropper to leading farmer—and now Floresta's loan officer in Haiti. And I have had the privilege of meeting and helping hundreds of people with similar stories."

Today Floresta works in three widely separated regions of Haiti, with a local staff of more than 20. Floresta agronomists teach the farmers to control erosion, incorporate trees into their farms, and increase their yields. Access to credit helps people use their initiative and avoid short-term crises. Training in Christian spiritual disciplines is the glue that holds all the work together. Floresta has shown that by helping the poor realize their God-given talents, they can shape a better future.

The organization's success continues to spread. In addition to Haiti, Floresta is helping thousands of villagers in Mexico, the Dominican Republic, Tanzania, and Thailand. Scott is quick to point out that reforestation programs will fail when local villagers have no sense of ownership for the forest. But thanks to Floresta, the vicious cycle of deforestation and poverty can become a virtuous cycle of reforestation and economic empowerment.

Since 1985, Floresta has helped plant 3.5 million trees, awarded hundreds of thousands of dollars in loans, and helped more than 25,000 people in 150 villages around the world. Volunteers are always welcome to accompany the staff when they visit rural villages. "At Floresta, we teach, we plant, we create enterprise, and we share the Gospel, all in an effort to transform lives," Scott said. "And anyone who wants to join me in putting out those fires is welcome."

For More Information

Save mountains, stop deforestation, plant trees, save lives, breathe easier. Contact today:

Floresta USA
4903 Morena Blvd, Suite 1215
San Diego, California 92117
Phone: (800) 633-5319
Website: www.floresta.org

Mark Stuart
Hands and Feet Project

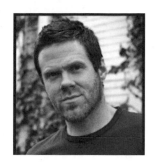

A Village to Raise & Love Abandoned Children

Mark Stuart, the lead singer of the internationally acclaimed rock band Audio Adrenaline, said his best day and worst day happened in the same 24-hour period, when the plight of a unknown girl, thousands of miles away and living a world apart from his affluent existence, broke his heart.

It was July 8, 2007. A 16-year-old Haitian girl had learned she was pregnant, and she didn't welcome the news. But she came up with a plan: She would give birth in a latrine and leave the child to die. When she went into labor, she left the baby girl lying at the bottom of a public toilet that was little more than a deep hole in the ground. Hearing the heartbreaking story of the girl and the baby she had left to die made July 8 Mark's worst day.

But something happened that the young mother hadn't counted on: A 14-year-old boy saw what happened. When the girl left, he went and looked into the toilet, where he saw the newborn at the bottom of the 30-foot-deep hole. He went to a United Nations office for help. The boy led adults to the latrine, where they were able to lift the baby to safety.

The next day, the child was taken to the Hands and Feet Project, a children's village started by Mark and his fellow Audio Adrenaline band members. While Mark wasn't in Haiti at the time, he heard about the rescue as it was happening and saw video of it that same day.

"This baby was reborn almost," Mark said. "She was wrapped in a sheet and pulled up by a rope. When my wife and I saw that, it was so emotional for us. That was the worst day—and the best." They were hooked and committed.

Now Mark and his wife sponsor the baby girl, who was named Christela. Their sponsorship provides all her financial needs—including food, caretakers, clothing, and medical care. Mark thinks of it as a financial adoption. "We look at her as our daughter," he said.

A year later, Christela is a bright-eyed, healthy baby with a big smile. She's one of about two dozen children in the Hands and Feet family. Though the children's village itself hasn't been around long, the origin of Hands and Feet goes back decades.

The story started when Mark was a child. His father, a pastor, frequently went on mission trips and would return with stories of adventure and God working in miraculous ways. Even as a young boy, Mark looked forward to going on a mission trip himself one day.

That dream was fulfilled when Mark was about 13 and his dad took him to Haiti, the poorest country in the Western Hemisphere. There Mark found a world far different from what he had always known in the United States.

"It was eye opening to see you don't have to have everything. You don't have to be completely comfortable," he said. "I knew at that point that Haiti would always be a passion."

The day after Mark graduated from high school, his parents moved to Haiti to serve as missionaries. Mark visited as much as possible, so often that Haiti felt like home. But it would be a while before his life would become wrapped up in Haiti because he spent the next 16 years of his life traveling the world with Audio Adrenaline.

While a college student, Mark and a couple of friends formed a band called A-180, and it was an instant success at their college in Kentucky. After graduation, the band morphed into Audio Adrenaline and released its first album in 1992. In the following years, they were nominated for 20 Dove Awards—and won four. They also won two Grammy Awards and had 18 No. 1 radio hits, including songs like "Big House," "Never Gonna Be As Big As Jesus," and "Hands and Feet."

Even as a young musician, Mark considered being a missionary, but on a trip to Haiti he sensed God telling him that instead he would get American young people involved in missions.

The band consistently encouraged its huge audiences to get involved in missions, even focusing an entire album, *Worldwide*, on the cause. But in 2004 they realized it was time to stop just challenging others to change the world. It was time to change the world themselves.

"I think that, as a band, we were served so much that one day we awoke to what was going on and said it was time for us to serve others," Mark recalled. Also, Mark's voice was wearing out after years of constant use as Audio Adrenaline's lead singer. They knew they couldn't keep the band going forever.

The band members decided to focus their missions work in Haiti, where they would start a children's village, where orphans' lives would be saved and they would have a loving, compassionate, Christian environment to grow up in. Mark's parents, Drex and Jo Stuart, would lead the project.

With the help of volunteer groups from the United States, the village was ready to open in 2006. They named the program Hands and Feet Project, drawing on a song of the same name Stuart wrote for Audio Adrenaline in the late 1990s. "I really wanted to empower people with that song—that you truly can make a difference in people's lives," Stuart said. "It's more than just about passing out tracts or preaching; it's about getting out there and becoming the hands of Jesus to touch people, the way he touched people."

The Hands and Feet village is just outside Jacmel, a city on Haiti's southern coast. The main building sits on three and a half acres of land. Blue rocking chairs line the front porch, and the building includes amenities found in few Haitian homes—electricity, running water, an oven, ceiling fans, and even Internet access. In addition to housing the children, caretakers, and staff, the building also is designed to house short-term mission volunteer teams. Eventually, the group plans to build smaller houses around the property to house more children and their caretakers.

The goal of Hands and Feet is to care for children no one else wants. By raising them in a loving, stable, Christian home, they believe these children will grow up to positively change the future of their impoverished country.

The first child taken in by Hands and Feet was Thamara. This little girl's mother died a few months after giving birth, and her father refused to care for her. She was malnourished when she was brought to Hands and Feet. At the time, the children's village's main building wasn't even finished, but the Stuarts couldn't let her go. They found a place for her with a nearby friend until the building was complete. Now Thamara is a chatty, cheery little girl with a big appetite, and she calls Hands and Feet home.

Mark and the other founders realize that one day the children of Hands and Feet—like Thamara and Christela—will grow up and might find themselves with no support system. "What's gonna happen when Christela turns 18?" Mark asks. "We see the gravity of the situation. They need to have opportunity to have their own families and provide for themselves."

So Hands and Feet is helping create industry in Haiti to provide sustainable incomes for the children who grow up at the children's village, as well as other Haitians. They're exploring ideas like starting a coffee plantation or goat farm, raising chickens, and developing a seamstresses' outpost. "To really make a dent in the Third World, we have to provide men and women the opportunity to pull themselves up with a sense of pride by their own bootstraps," Mark said.

Mark's vision ranges beyond Audio Adrenaline and Haiti. In 2006, Audio Adrenaline released its last album, *Adios*. Now they are expanding Hands and Feet into other countries and through other Christian bands. They have set their sights on Nicaragua—the second poorest country in the Western Hemisphere—as the next place the Hands and Feet model will be implemented.

As Audio Adrenaline works with younger bands, Mark thinks of himself as more of a big brother than a mentor. As bands work hard to put albums out, the members also want to make a practical difference in the world. Mark and Audio Adrenaline help them know how to do that. Through those partnerships, Mark hopes to use the power of celebrity to educate American churches and philanthropists about giving people a way out of poverty.

With Audio Adrenaline officially disbanded, Mark doesn't know exactly where the next 15 or 20 years of his life will lead, but he knows it will be far better than anything he could imagine. "We're all chosen for a reason, and despite what we consider our shortcomings, God can do great things through each of us," he said. "There's an abundant life out there. Ask him to do great things in your life. He'll show up and do beyond what you can imagine."

The Hands and Feet Project was started by Mark Stuart and Audio Adrenaline in 2004 when they purchased land to establish a village for abandoned children. They began construction in early 2005, and their first little girl arrived in the spring of that year. By 2007, more than 30 children ranging in age from 2 months to 9 years old live in the Hands and Feet children's village near Jacmel, Haiti.

The mission of Hands and Feet is two-fold—first, to care for orphans and, second, to use pop culture to introduce the First World to the orphans of the Third World. Their vision is to raise a generation of orphans raised within their own cultures who will, in turn, change their countries so orphanages are empty and Hands and Feet is out of a job. As the number of abandoned children is expected to grow to 40 in 2008, Hands and Feet plans to replicate the model next in Nicaragua, bringing artists and bands together with orphans.

For $125 a month, an individual can sponsor a child, covering everything the child needs—including food, education, caretakers, clothing, medical care, water, and utilities. Additionally, volunteers are welcomed at the children's village. Groups of up to 12 can stay at the children's village, helping with construction and spending time with the children.

Sing it loud with Mark ≈ Get involved to help build a village for our children. Connect with:

The Hands and Feet Project
PO Box 682105
Franklin, Tennessee 37068
Phone: (615) 550-4389
E-mail: info@hafproject.org
Website: www.handsandfeetproject.org

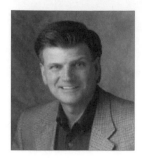

Franklin Graham
Samaritan's Purse

Charting a Different
Course from Dad

"Just being the son of Billy Graham won't get me into heaven."

–Franklin Graham, 1996

As 9-year-old Emily Nannyonjo unwrapped her present, her eyes flashed with unexpected joy. "I have never received a gift like this. I am so happy that God loves me," she said.

The gift was a simple shoebox, crammed with a small teddy bear, costume jewelry, school supplies, a personal note and a photo from Lesley Clementi, a 13-year-old girl in Florida. It was a gift from one HIV-positive girl to another.

Operation Christmas Child brought the two together.

More than seven million smiles—that's how many brightly wrapped shoeboxes packed with gifts were given to children like Emily in dire situations around the world this past Christmas. When a child who lives in a slum—a child who has never had a gift of any kind before—receives a box filled with presents, you have that child's attention. Operation Christmas Child creates an opportunity to tell that child about Christmas and about celebrating the birth of Jesus Christ.

More amazing than the impact of this compassionate giving is the inspiration for it all: a one-time hard-drinking, cigarette-smoking, party-hearty rebel with a family name he wasn't prepared to live up to.

Franklin Graham

Born in 1952, Franklin Graham was the fourth of five children of renowned evangelist Billy Graham and his wife, Ruth Bell Graham. Young Franklin was raised in the Appalachian Mountains outside Asheville, North Carolina.

For much of Franklin's early life, walking in his father's footsteps was the furthest thing from his mind; but in his book, *Rebel With A Cause*, Franklin describes a sleepless night in a Jerusalem hotel at the age of 22 when he had a spiritual awakening. "Suddenly, I was overcome with a conviction that I needed to get my life right with God," Franklin wrote. "I asked him to forgive me and come into my heart. By morning, my years of rebellion had ended."

Shortly after that epiphany, Franklin returned to North Carolina and married a hometown girl, Jane Austin Cunningham. The ceremony took place on his parents' front lawn, where he publicly told everyone how his life had changed. Franklin began looking for ways to show his faith.

In October 1975, a family friend, Dr. Bob Pierce, the founder of Samaritan's Purse and World Vision, invited young Graham to join him on a six-week mission to Asia. There, Franklin was overwhelmed by the raw hardships endured by so many of the world's poorest people. The black sheep of the Graham family knew he had found his direction.

Samaritan's Purse became the rebel's new cause. A nondenominational Christian organization providing spiritual and physical aid to the world's impoverished, this organization has met the needs of victims of war, poverty, natural disasters, disease and famine since 1970. "Samaritan's Purse is an evangelistic group that just happens to provide relief," Franklin said. "I'm not going to waste my time going around the world just doing 'do-good' things. Anybody can do 'do-good things.' I'm going to 'do-good things' with the Gospel."

In his early years with Samaritan's Purse, Franklin visited a number of hot spots around the globe. After Bob Pierce died of leukemia in 1978, Franklin Graham accepted the role of president and chairman. He was just 27 years old.

In that same year, two surgeon brothers, Lowell and Richard Furman, approached Franklin with a desire to volunteer for a short-term assignment in a mission hospital during their vacation. Franklin looked for other organizations already involved in that type of work, but to his surprise, there were none—so he helped the Furmans start World Medical Mission (WMM).

As a subsidiary of Samaritan's Purse, WMM assists hospitals and clinics in Africa, Asia, Latin America, and the Middle East. Every year, they send hundreds of volunteer physicians like the Furman brothers on short-term assignments to dozens of hospitals and clinics around the world. World Medical Mission also provides mission hospitals with critically needed supplies, equipment, and technical support.

Under Franklin's stewardship, Samaritan's Purse has grown into a $287 million organization, ranked in the top 50 U.S. nonprofits and efficiently spending only 11% of income on administration and fundraising.

Operation Christmas Child

In June of 1993, Franklin was working with Samaritan's Purse when he received a request from a man in England to help collect Christmas gift boxes for the children of war-ravaged Bosnia. "When he called again in November, I had completely forgotten about it," Franklin recalled. "So I went to one church and asked if they could fill 3,000 or 4,000 empty shoeboxes with little gifts and toys. By mid-week, the church had called to ask if someone could *please* come and get the boxes that were stacked everywhere. That one community had collected 11,000 shoeboxes."

"Every box given by a family is like a snowflake—there aren't two the same...In 2007, we delivered gifts to 7.5 million children in over 100 countries."

Handing out the gifts in Bosnia, Franklin realized the opportunities for Samaritan's Purse to touch the lives of children throughout the world were limitless. Inspired by the joy with which the Bosnian children received the gifts, he took it one step further and created Operation Christmas Child. "Every box given by a family is like a snowflake—there aren't two the same," he said. "The families pray for the children who receive the boxes. We started with 11,000 shoeboxes packed with gifts, love and prayers. In 2007, we delivered gifts to 7.5 million children in over 100 countries." Over the years, these small packages have brought not only joy, but also the true meaning of Christmas—Jesus Christ.

While Franklin continued to minister through Samaritan's Purse and Operation Christmas Child, his father was beginning to consider the need to name a successor for the Billy Graham Evangelistic Association (BGEA). Though he was in his eighties, the elder Graham still was packing stadiums and thousands of lives were being changed through his preaching. People urged Franklin to pick up the mantle of his father's legacy, including following him into the pulpit. For years he resisted. "Evangelistic preaching is what Daddy does; I never thought I would," Franklin said. However, Franklin ultimately did begin leading evangelistic festivals under the BGEA. Then in 2000 he became the head of BGEA while remaining president of Samaritan's Purse. "I've now got two jobs," he said, "I love them both."

Today Franklin and his wife, Jane, live on a farm in Boone, North Carolina. He travels a great deal with his work, but makes a point of not staying away from his family for too long. He has long since abandoned the drinking, smoking, and partying habits of his youth, but he retains one last element of his "wild" side—an occasional motorcycle ride on the winding mountain roads of western North Carolina. It's all the high he needs these days.

With a name like Graham, it's difficult to avoid the national spotlight. Franklin preached at the memorial service for victims of the Columbine High School shooting and at the funeral of musician Johnny Cash. He also delivered the invocation at President George W. Bush's inauguration in January 2001.

Once reluctant to follow in his father's footsteps, Graham is now thankful for his role. He has made his own mark on the world, including the joy that lights up the faces of millions of children in Third World countries. "I've been called to the slums of the streets and the ditches of the world. I just want to be faithful to the same message that my dad's been faithful to," he said, "And that's the preaching of the Gospel."

Samaritan's Purse travels the highways of the world looking for victims along the way. The work is often dangerous—as it was for the Good Samaritan—but the message they carry is much too important. Quick to bandage the wounds they see, these Samaritans don't stop there. In addition to the work of Operation Christmas Child and World Medical Mission, Samaritan's Purse provides disaster relief and assistance in more than 100 countries around the world. Projects include rebuilding hundreds of churches destroyed by civil war in Sudan, feeding over 100,000 refugees in Darfur, and providing housing for thousands of families affected by the tsunami in South Asia and Hurricane Katrina.

Over the past 15 years, Operation Christmas Child has delivered more than 60 million gift-filled shoeboxes to hurting children around the world.

Create Christ-filled Christmas gift boxes and support Samaritan's Purse. Contact:

Samaritan's Purse

PO Box 3000

Boone, NC 28607

Phone: (828) 262-1980 | Fax: (828) 266-1053

Website: www.samaritanspurse.org

Operation Christmas Child

Phone: (800) 353-5949

E-mail: occinfo@samaritan.org

CELEBRATING PASSIONARIES
FOR HUMANITY

"We have every right to dream heroic dreams.
Those who say that we're in a time
when there are no heroes,
they just don't know where to look."
—Ronald Reagan, January 20, 1981

"Hope lives in dreams,
in imagination,
and in the courage of those
who demand
to make dreams into reality."
—Jonas Salk

"Everyone can be great,
because everyone can serve."
—Martin Luther King, Jr.

"Many persons have a wrong idea
of what constitutes true happiness.
It is not attained through self-gratification
but through fidelity to a worthy purpose."
—Helen Keller

John van Hengel
Feeding America

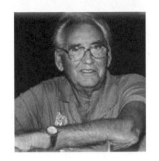

Food Banks for the Hungry

It was not a sudden epiphany that changed John van Hengel's priorities and passions, but rather an endless string of observations and worrisome questions. *How*, in the richest, best-fed, fattest nation in the world, could millions of adults and children go hungry for several days each month? How could the enormous waste in America's food industry be redirected to help people in need?

That was in 1967, when John was living in Phoenix, reduced to wearing rags, struggling to find purpose after squandering the rich opportunity of a promising young life. During the last three decades of his life, John took a vow of poverty and in the beginning lived on very little. He worked his first 10 years with St. Mary's Food Bank without salary. He ate Spam from unlabeled cans on two-day-old rolls. The clothes he wore came from Salvation Army bins. His home was a donated room above a garage.

> *"How, in the richest, best-fed, fattest nation in the world, could millions of adults and children go hungry for several days each month?"*

John was, in part, adhering to the vows of personal poverty followed by another feeder of the lost: Mother Teresa. In every way, he actively pursued his belief in the Bible, particularly Matthew 6:19, "Lay not up for yourselves treasures upon earth...but lay up for yourselves treasures in heaven...for where your treasure is, there will your heart be also."

Even at age 78, faltering from several strokes as well as the first toll of Parkinson's Disease, John still had his treasure securely banked in heaven. His small consulting fee from the food bank, lumped with a Social Security check, totaled the humble sum of $12,000 per year. That was enough for toothpaste, a telephone, and the rent for a one-bedroom cube of an apartment cluttered with second-hand furniture. His wardrobe consisted of whatever anyone gave him that fit. All of it was a world away from the Beverly Hills playboy van Hengel had once been.

Born to a Dutch-American family of physicians, nurses, and pharmacists who lived well and problem-free in Wisconsin, John left Lawrence University in 1944 with a degree in government. A football injury kept him out of World War II, but not off intercollegiate tennis courts and the road to Southern California.

"I found I liked the good life and became a first-rate beach bum," he once recalled. He played volleyball at Muscle Beach and tennis at the Beverly Wilshire Hotel. He also got a job with Ben Pollack, a big band leader who became an agent. Pollack's clients were Kay Starr and Mel Torme; John's were the jugglers and strippers.

In time, John regained his focus. He studied broadcasting at UCLA and started on a series of careers, becoming, in turn, a magazine publicist, a garment industry ad man, a designer of plastic rainwear, and a maitre d' in a restaurant. When he married an I. Magnin model, it seemed there would be no looking back. Then, in 1960, the couple divorced.

"I took off back to Wisconsin, hurt, escaping and so angry that I wanted the worst job I could find," John remembered. "I went to work in a quarry making rocks with a sledgehammer and a pick. Our gang was ornery and mean. Anybody working in a quarry didn't have much going for him. Neither did I."

Then John was injured in a factory fight, and a spinal surgery left him with a locked neck, palsy, and bad legs. Told his recovery would go better in a warmer, drier climate, he arrived in Phoenix with a few dollars and no job. Endless laps in a YMCA pool brought strength back to his body. He drove a school bus and advanced to city employee. "At 44, I was the oldest public pools lifeguard in Phoenix," he said.

Along the way, John also found new spiritual strength, but not from any conscious searching. He started reading the Bible as a primer for attending a Franciscan retreat where the brothers showed movies about world hunger. "As I read, I realized I was doing the things I should be doing...my work was following what was written in the Bible," John said.

That "work" was helping with a charity dining room and recovering out-of-date collection cans donated from grocery stores. His salary was 30% of the loose change. John also befriended alcoholics and helped the helpless. Starting out with an antiquated ex-milk truck he bought for $150, he picked surplus oranges, lemons, and grapefruit from homeowners' trees and hauled the fruit to charity missions.

Then John started looking for a place to store the citrus and found an abandoned bakery that had been willed to the Franciscans of St. Mary's Basilica, close to where the needy huddled on Skid Row. The parish council even chipped in $3,000 for a telephone, utilities, and the conversion of the bakery's hot room into a cool room for the fruit.

Everything came together late in 1967, when a city social worker introduced John to a woman who had 10 children, and a husband on death row. She told him that, even with her dire circumstances, finding food was no problem. She did her daily shopping in refuse bins behind a nearby grocery store.

John went to the bins himself. "I found frozen food that had been thrown out but was still frozen, still edible," he said. "Loose carrots. Stale bread." The store manager showed him less perishable leavings in a back room: a case of ketchup condemned by one broken bottle. Bags leaking rice and sugar from small tears. A dozen dented cans and many more "shiners"—cans without labels.

The manager said everything would be thrown out. John asked if he could take it for the hungry. When the manager agreed, John made the same pitch with other grocery managers. The old bakery began to bulge. A friend who had volunteered to help, drew a cartoon of food being deposited and happy people making withdrawals. Just like a bank. Van Hengel roared: "That's it! We'll call this place St. Mary's Food Bank!"

In that first year, after spreading the scrounging to Tucson, Prescott, Yuma, and Flagstaff, St. Mary's Food Bank distributed more than 250,000 pounds of food including 5,000 live chickens, 500 cases of anchovies, and, in a unique agreement with a friendly judge, 539,000 gallons of milk to 36 charities—part of a sentence against local dairies convicted of price fixing.

The St. Mary's example inspired the Grandview Bank of Pasadena, the nation's second food bank. Others followed in San Diego, San Jose, and Concord. Then Portland and Seattle.

"It all just fell into place, step-by-step," John recalled. "The evolution was there and the potential unbelievable. But I can't really claim fatherhood. It was the will of the good Lord. I just plodded. If the door opened, I went in. If the door closed, I backed off and started again."

Eventually, John found most of his answers. His dream of a national network of food banks gave rise to two organizations: St. Mary's Food Bank and Feeding America (formerly America's Second Harvest), the nation's food bank network. These two groups, which he founded with nothing more than a dilapidated truck and a vision, flourished instantly and today help feed 25 million hungry people every year.

Going beyond domestic hunger needs, John also started Food Banking International to address hunger issues across the globe. His vision for food banking in other countries has now been realized in the formation of the Global FoodBanking Network with sites in Africa, Japan, and South America.

Each day, volunteers inspired by John's simple dream attack hunger in the pinched, crowded corners of cities like Los Angeles, New York, and Detroit, where they offload hundreds of tractor-trailers laden with groceries. Some, like the brown pouches and olive-drab cans, came from a $300 million government food surplus. Others, like 37 railroad cars of cereal with too many raisins and 5 million pounds of ravioli not cooked to company standards, came from generous food distributors.

In the desert city of Phoenix stands the monument to the history and ingenuity of it all—the original St. Mary's Food Bank, built in an abandoned bakery in a dying barrio. Ten years ago, the organization expanded into a 120,000 square-foot warehouse in West Phoenix, a structure requiring computerized logistics, fueled by an annual budget in the millions. As the source of 200,000 meals a day, and a paid executive who answers to an impressive board of directors, St. Mary's is the inspiration for offshoots around the world.

"We have certainly come a long way from when John started the food bank so many years ago," said Cynde Cerf, director of community relations for St. Mary's Food Bank Alliance. "Processes are more complex and we have to be much more creative when working with donors. However, the basic concept is still the same. We are here to feed people, provide them with a basic need. This is something of which John always reminded me. It is the driving force behind our mission every day."

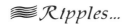

In 1976, John van Hengel left St. Mary's Food Bank to birth Feedng America (formerly America's Second Harvest). First based in Phoenix and funded by a $50,000 federal grant, Feeding America counseled cities wanting to establish food banks. It also tapped into food disposal programs at the manufacturing level. Today, Feeding America is a network of 205 food banks, which in turn provide food and grocery products to more than 50,000 food pantries, soup kitchens, inner city missions, and other emergency feeding centers.

Feeding America's statistics are staggering: More than 2 billion pounds of food and grocery products are distributed each year, feeding 25 million Americans, including 9 million children and 3 million senior adults. The organization has a 98% efficiency rating. Across America, more than 1 million volunteers give their time to feed the hungry through Feeding America.

At its heart, the organization actually is an assault on hunger and a secondary welfare system managed by the private sector in more than 200 American cities. There also are eight major food banks in Canada, 74 in France, nine in Belgium, 35 in Italy, and others in Ireland, Spain, Australia, and Israel.

When America's Second Harvest moved to Chicago, operations soon became entangled in bureaucracy. It was no place for people who did business on a handshake. So John quit in 1983 and returned to his roots in Phoenix, where he remained available to anyone with a storefront and dreams of feeding the poor.

"It is amazing how many people are being fed because of this crazy little thing we started," John once said. The collective pronoun "we" included his original staff: a Latina grandmother and two physically challenged volunteers. "We're feeding millions, and it is not costing anyone anything," he said. "But it scares me to look back, because I just had no idea it would grow into this."

Oddly, John was not the only van Hengel who made such a contribution. Years ago, traveling on a tourist ticket that had been given to him (of course!), John visited his Dutch relatives in Amsterdam. Visiting family gravesites in a country cemetery near the city, he found the grave of a forebear who had died in 1649. The epitaph on Dirk van Hengel's gravestone read: "He fed the poor of Germany."

John died peacefully in 2005 at the age of 83—furthering the van Hengel golden legacy of feeding the poor.

North County Food Bank, San Marcos, California

After a 26 year military career, Mike Doody's first civilian position was director of the San Diego Food Bank—a large and very unstable program. "In 2003, I met John van Hengel at a Second Harvest conference. This simple man decided to do something helpful for others and it multiplied into the amazing network of Food Banks throughout America," reflected Mike. "Interestingly, each one was uniquely different in how they provide emergency food for the needy." In 2005, Mike transitioned to the much smaller North County Food Bank where he put into practice the ideals of John Van Hengel.

"First I began to develop partnerships with grocery stores and food purveyors. I began to attend community fairs and volunteer associated events to develop partnerships with schools and community colleges that encouraged community service at the local level." In 2007, this began to pay dividends. Two high school seniors elected to have their senior project be a food distribution point in their deprived neighborhoods. This continues to be a tremendously successful community serving effort.

In total, North County Food Bank has grown from serving 9,500 people in need to more than 15,500 people each month, partnering with 75 various agencies. His program averages 50-60 individual volunteers serving over 800 volunteer hours each month. "Since I started in North County, our food distributions have soared from 440,000 pounds per year to exceeding 1.2 million pounds!"

During Mike's 2007 term as President of his local Optimist Club of Carlsbad, he helped establish a joint partnership to do semi-annual food drives. In addition to other programs, Optimist volunteers prepare two dinner meals for hungry people each month. The alliance between The Optimist Club and North County Food Bank continues to pay big dividends for both groups.

Kids Café

In Savannah, Georgia in 1989, two young brothers were discovered late one night in the kitchen of their housing project's community center. The older brother had broken into the kitchen to feed himself and his younger brother. In response to this glaring example of childhood hunger in their community, The Second Harvest Food Bank of Coastal Georgia started the first Kids Café. In 1993, America's Second Harvest launched the national Kids Café program. By 2007, more than 1,600 Kids Café sites were in operation.

In Phoenix alone, The Kids Café at St. Mary's Food Bank provides food to 25 sites. Serving as many as 1,800 meals daily, their dedicated volunteers provide more than 400,000 meals to low-income children ages 5 to 18, usually in conjunction with after-school programs. They work in partnership with area churches, schools, community centers, Boys and Girls Clubs of America, and city parks and recreation departments to help provide food and a secure and safe environment for children.

Community Kitchens

Community Kitchens was founded in 1989 by Robert Egger with DC Central Kitchen. The program expanded into a national program with the nonprofit organization Food Chain in 1997 and then became a Feeding America/America's Second Harvest national program with the merging of the two nonprofits in 2000. There are currently 18 active Community Kitchens in the Feeding America network.

These Community Kitchen programs provide culinary job training to low-income men and women to prepare them for careers in the food service industry. The students who often struggle to find a job due to unfortunate circumstances in their background, enroll in a 16-week training to prepare food. While in the program, they also develop valuable life and professional skills including goal establishment, resumé writing, interviewing skills, conflict management and budgeting to help them gain and sustain employment after graduation.

As the students work to achieve their own self-sufficiency, they also serve their communities, producing hundreds of nutritious meals for a variety of social service agency feeding programs such as Kids Cafes, youth and senior centers, shelters and community dining rooms. With

21 different Community Kitchen programs nationwide, by 2006 this innovative program had more than 1,100 students in training and served 4.7 million meals. Their students are trained and directed to find employment in the foodservice industry.

The Community Kitchen program is an innovative, exciting, and cost-efficient way to feed the hungry, train the unemployed, generate public support, create greater economies of scale, and challenge inaccurate stereotypes of the men, women, and children served.

For more information about Community Kitchen programs, please contact Mitzi Baum at (312) 641-6842 or at mbaum@secondharvest.org.

For More Information

John van Hengel originated the concept of food banks, creating St. Mary's Food Bank in Phoenix in 1967. He helped start food banks in many other locations, and now almost every city in America and around the world can claim one.

In 1976, John van Hengel left St. Mary's and started Feeding America, which now helps feed more than 25 million Americans every year, including 9 million children and 3 million senior adults. A total of 50,000 local relief agencies partner with 500 national grocery chains and food companies to help hungry people. One in four people in a soup kitchen line is a child. Across America, more than 1 million volunteers annually give their time to feed the hungry through Feeding America, not counting international volunteers.

Help the harvest for people in need of food and bank on making a difference. Call:

Feeding America
35 East Wacker Drive, #2000, Chicago, Illinois 60601
Phone: (800) 771-2303
Website: www.secondharvest.org/foodbanks/locator.html

St. Mary's Food Bank Alliance
2831 North 31st Avenue, Phoenix, Arizona 85009-1415
Phone: (602) 352-3640 | Fax: (602) 352-3659
Website: www.firstfoodbank.org
To get the latest facts about this issue, visit:
www.hungerinamerica.org.

Bob McElroy
Alpha Project for the Homeless

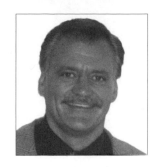

Where Miracles Happen!

Opportunities, not Handouts, for the Homeless

"Bag ladies, dumpster divers, bums, panhandlers, dope fiends—that's what the public usually thinks of when you mention the homeless," said Bob McElroy, president and CEO of The Alpha Project in San Diego. "They believe these people are worth no more than shelters offer them: 'three hots and a cot.'"

Since 1986, Bob and his Alpha Project team have been proving the skeptics wrong. Time and time again, they have demonstrated that when people living on the streets are given opportunities and support, they become community assets rather than liabilities. By offering the homeless a fresh start, respect, and self-determination—rather than handouts, pity, and control—Alpha Project enables homeless people to end the cycle of dependence that prevents them from enjoying a life of dignity.

Alpha Project enables homeless people to end the cycle of dependence that prevents them from enjoying a life of dignity.

Despite his opinion about handouts, Bob started his project with a handout. "I was feeding people with my church group in San Diego's Balboa Park on Friday nights," Bob said. "I was a minister at the time, bragging to friends about the warm fuzzies I was getting by saving these people for Jesus. But I saw that if I didn't bring sandwiches, they would lie around drinking beer, doing drugs, panhandling or engaging in prostitution. And then the light bulb went on: I wasn't really helping anyone."

With a bedroll tucked under his arm, Bob decided to spend 10 weeks living in the park with the homeless. He was one of the first to hold up a "Will work for food" sign—but he never had to make good on the offer. "There were 17 other churches and do-gooder groups coming down there to feed people," he said. "In the summertime, Balboa Park is beautiful; it became an urban campground with a party atmosphere. People were using their welfare checks to hold keg parties. Charitable groups gave us jackets, nice clothing, blankets, and sleeping bags. We had swap meets in the park because you could only carry around so much of what was donated.

"For many of these folks, it was all a game and they'd laugh about the lifestyle: 'Hey, we don't have to do anything and can get cash just by begging. We can get all the drugs and alcohol we want and people bring down big buffet dinners for us.' It was a rude awakening for me that I had been part of the problem instead of part of the solution."

At the end of his experiment, Bob packed up his sleeping bag and stopped in to talk about the situation with the businesses that ringed the park. One of them offered him a small office to use as a base of operations. Before developing a strategy, however, Bob felt he had to understand the root of the problem. Nobody started out in life on the streets or working as a prostitute. Each evening for the next two years, he brought in homeless people, one or two at a time, and talked with them. Why were they there? What was going on in their life?

To be of any help to the homeless, Bob realized that the first thing he'd have to do was get them into legitimate regular employment. The next step was turning his cramped office space into a makeshift employment agency. A nearby restaurant hired two of Bob's new friends as cooks, and other businesses passed along job opportunities. Soon, hardcore gang members, chronic homeless people, and drug addicts were heading off to work each morning and came back to the park at night to sleep.

The first big break, however, came when the owner of a chain of steak houses bought a long-abandoned building adjacent to Balboa Park. Bob hired up to 50 homeless people a day, first to tear down the old structure and then to build the new one. The project attracted media attention, and soon neighboring cities were contacting Bob to create programs for their homeless.

It was then that Bob came face to face with another hard reality. "Finding jobs for people was easy," he said. "But I soon learned that it wasn't bad luck that had gotten them to where they were; it was bad choices. I would send people out to work. They would work for two weeks until they got their first paycheck. Then they would disappear for three days, blow their whole paycheck, and come back. I realized I had to deal with their core issues, whether it was lying, addiction, manipulation, fraud, or conning people."

To maintain credibility with employers, Bob went to the "work crew" concept. With funding support from churches and organizations, he put homeless people to work for the Alpha Project and then contracted them out to other employers as work crews. Bob said, "That's what we have done ever since and it works." The concept is that those who are able-bodied and can work, will work for Alpha Project first, learn the basics—staying sober, getting up every morning prepared to be an asset, paying bills, building positive relationships, etc. Then, after they have acquired the basic skills, they are ready to transition into an outside job.

"At our kick-off fundraiser, a women's group adopted me and Alpha Project. We generated enough money to buy our first truck so we could take on bigger jobs. These women hired my guys—who were hardcore, ex-convict gang members, chronic homeless people, and drug addicts—to escort them safely at night from their small downtown businesses to their cars," Bob chuckles.

Each year Alpha Project programs serve more than 12,000 homeless and very-low income people and families in communities from Riverside to Chula Vista in Southern California. Conceived as a simple initiative offering work opportunities for homeless men, the Alpha Project now operates 16 programs across six cities and two counties. The agency grew into providing emergency housing, outreach, HIV/ AIDS services, supportive housing for the mentally ill and infirmed, residential treatment for the addicted, and hospice care. Additionally, they have created affordable rental housing projects and sponsored home ownership programs. In 1990, President George H. W. Bush gave national recognition to Bob's work by honoring him as a "Point of Light."

The Alpha Project is not a "bed and breakfast" organization. "We're not a shelter," Bob said. "People have to work—they have to commit. You can't just lie around for two years, be fed, and attend a few classes."

Getting people off drugs is never easy, but Bob and his volunteers have a fine track record with that challenge, too. "One year after graduating from our program, 82% of the participants are still clean and sober. Compare that to a national average of about 26%," Bob said. "We don't dictate to people. We have a program, and they must partner in it. There are no fences or dogs. They can leave at any time."

These days, on any given morning on many of the main streets of North San Diego County, smiling men stand at intersections, waving newspapers for sale. Their friendly faces and comic antics make drivers want to stop and buy a paper, even though newspapers are sitting unread on their front porches at home. As much as selling papers, these once destitute drug addicts have found they *want* to make people start their day with a smile. The income from the newspapers they sell supports the drug clinics where they live.

The program may be working, but final success to Bob McElroy means going out of business—no more homeless people needing help. "There are plenty of other causes," he said. "I started out wanting to do something for homeless children. But you can't give children a nurturing, supportive environment during the day and then send them home to a street corner or parents on drugs. I figured we would solve the parents issue first, and then get around to the kids."

On any given day, 2,000 people are involved in the program. "We have 700 families in our permanent housing and a seniors' facility in Vista with 92 units," Bob said. "Computers and computer instruction are available for kids whose families can't afford them. One of our facilities is located in an Hispanic area, so the staff tutors children in English as a second language. We also operate shuttle buses that take people to their appointments, especially at our seniors' facility. And we have a special van that provides medical outreach treatment for homeless kids."

In 1991, at the invitation of the City of San Diego, the Alpha Project began operating the Neil Good Day Center, the city's only full-service day center for homeless people. More than 400 homeless men, women, and children use the center each day for showers, social service referrals, mail and message service, laundry facilities, safe storage, mental health counseling, substance abuse recovery meetings, and job opportunities. Additionally, Alpha Project operated the City's Winter Shelter for homeless men and women.

Bob thinks that if Jesus walked into Balboa Park, he also would focus on giving people opportunities to change their lives. "It's your responsibility to have a relationship with your Maker," Bob said. "I can't force you to do that. I'm a Christian minister who wasn't called to be a pastor. I'm in what you call 'application ministry.' Jesus didn't tell people to build him a marble sanctuary. He was down where I am, in the park and on the streets."

Bob believes in making your own reality, but he also knows a little about divine intervention. "I met my wife over the telephone," he said. "She worked at the bank and I was overdrawn, so she had to call me every day. She knew I didn't have any money, but she liked me anyway. That's the basis of everything for me. As they say, 'the rest is history.'"

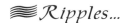 *Ripples...*

Joel Myers

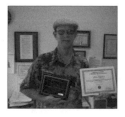

In April 2001, Martin Luther King III toured the Alpha Project's programs. King's visit was particularly special because three men were about to graduate from a year-long journey to a new life of hope and recovery.

One of them was Joel Myers, whose graduation was especially emotional because his mother, Evelyn, and his siblings, Mary and Jay, had traveled all the way from Georgia to honor his achievement. During the ceremony, Joel tearfully told his mother he had finally finished something that he had started—other than a bottle of booze.

Since Joel's graduation, he has been awarded the first Employee of the Quarter Award at Casa Raphael which is one of Alpha Project's two residential treatment programs for homeless men in recovery. He also was selected to attend the California Association of Addiction Recovery Resources program and finished his training and certification at the top of his class. He was immediately hired as an intern case manager and eventually was promoted to program manager.

"The best case managers," Bob McElroy said, "are those who can sit on the other side of a desk and relate to a person who walks through the door seeking help. Nearly all our staff are people who have been there, done that. That's why we are successful."

Since 1986, Bob McElroy's Alpha Project has shown that when down-and-out people are given opportunities and support, many of them become community assets, rather than liabilities. Numbers tell just part of the story. Every day, the Alpha Project's programs serve more than 2,000 homeless people. More than 12,000 different men, women, and children access one or more of their services each year. Their newest program launched in 2006, responds to the high mortality rate among the homeless. Their Hospice for the Homeless program provides assistance to veterans, homeless people, and indigent people facing terminal or chronic illness.

If your heart beats for the homeless, help make miracles happen. Contact:

Alpha Project for the Homeless

3737 Fifth Avenue, Suite 203

San Diego, California 92103

Phone: (619) 542-1877

E-mail: info@alphaproject.org

Website: www.alphaproject.org

*"Nothing great in the world
has been accomplished
without passion."*
—Georg Wilhelm

Prison Fellowship

These following three profiles are ripples of Chuck Colson's Prison Fellowship, the most effective rehabilitative national and international organization serving the 2 million people and their families who are in United States prisons today.

Catherine Rohr
Prison Entrepreneurship Program

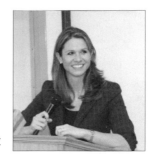

Connecting Ideas from the Inside Out

In 2003, as 26-year-old, model-gorgeous venture capitalist, Catherine Rohr sat in her Manhattan apartment, she could never have anticipated that her future would be behind bars—voluntarily—in a Texas men's prison. How Catherine made this life transition, and the effects of her compassion on Texas criminals, is a story worthy of a feature movie.

Everything in Catherine Rohr's training pointed toward success: loving family, excellent education, supportive spouse, and the aptitude to compete and succeed in the world of private equity and high finance. Her newly minted Christian heart led her and her husband to take a mission trip to Romania where they worked with HIV orphans, face-to-face with third-world injustice and heartbreak. Returning from Romania, she felt restless and disturbed that her life was so centered on her own comfort and personal success.

A year later, a woman friend invited Catherine to go to Texas on an Easter-time prison tour with Chuck Colson and Prison Fellowship. Catherine recalled saying, "What's a chick like you doing in a prison with a bunch of inmates?" When her friend shared her passion to help prisoners, Catherine was intrigued and challenged. She and her husband decided to cancel plans for a trip to California and go to Texas instead.

Every expectation they had was negative. What they had seen in the movies painted prison as the ultimate bad news industry. Since she had completely written off the entire prison population as being in the "bad pile," she expected to see caged animals. She recalled the ugliness in her heart: "Lock them up and throw away the key, they're taking up tax dollars." Catherine was surprised when she met real human beings who challenged her beliefs. She was shocked to learn that one out of every 15 Americans do prison time. And she realized that God loves these people, too.

As a venture capitalist, Catherine was trained to recognize opportunity and talent. She had conversations with dope dealers and gang leaders. From these interactions she learned that gangs are run by boards of directors and have commissioned sales structures and bookkeepers. They understand distribution channels and risk management. She heard tales of $100,000 in sales per week, 90% net margins, 90% repeat business. A company like that would have generated widespread interest in the investment community—had the core product not been crack cocaine. And the men certainly understood concepts like execution!

Catherine learned that the biggest missing link for criminals is that they usually didn't have a father or, if they did, wished they didn't have one. So many of them were raised in a destructive family cycle where crime is the norm and prison its natural consequence. She recalled wondering how much potential these men might have had, if they just had positive role models to show them how to live.

"It was like breathing life into these prisoners to tell them they don't have to live this life of crime, that there are legitimate ways to make it, and that God had a bigger plan for them."

The following month, Catherine had to travel back to Texas for a friend's wedding and decided to go by the prison again to teach the prisoners a little about what she knew best: business. She recruited a few executives to come with her saying, "Fly out to Texas with me in two weeks, and we will put on a Business 101 panel for two hours in prison." Three brave executives said, "yes!" Two of the three CEOs who taught the class to 55 convicts actually cried. "It was like breathing life into these prisoners to tell them they don't have to live this life of crime, that there are legitimate ways to make it, and that God had a bigger plan for them," Catherine added. "We told them they are not trash and they don't need to be just like their daddy."

Catherine was so moved during this class that she stood up at the end and said: "OK, we're going to start a business plan competition, right here, right now. And your first assignment is due next week." Had she realized the challenges of working in prison, she may have never taken on this project.

Back in her comfortable New York apartment with her lawyer husband, Catherine started corresponding with "her guys" and began flying out to Texas each month to teach them business skills. "Her guys" became Catherine's consuming passion. She explained why her heart was touched: "The criminal system releases these men with $100 and the clothes on their backs. How can we expect them to make it when you can't even get a job at Wal-Mart or flip burgers at McDonald's if you're a felon? Convicted felons are the most discriminated-against people in our country."

Catherine and her husband decided to jump ship, they gave up their jobs and moved to Texas. "This was a journey of saying 'Yes, God, yes, God' when the prayer up until then had been 'Bring it on,'" Catherine shares. "That was dangerous, because that kind of prayer can lead you to Texas!" Shortly after moving, they went broke and got robbed. It was a case of losing it all, then gaining everything.

Prison Entrepreneurship Program (PEP) was created by Catherine in 2004 for inmates nearing release. It is very challenging to be accepted into the program. The application process is purposely arduous to weed out "perverts and slackers." Those who are accepted spend 24 hours a week in the classroom, plus homework. They have a hunger to learn and grow and really show what they can do. Business people and MBA students come into the prison each week during the four-month class to mentor these dedicated prisoners.

Upon release, PEP provides job placement services, housing assistance, executive mentoring, continued education, and a large dose of accountability. More than 600,000 prisoners are released in the U.S. each year, with two-thirds returning to the criminal justice system within two to three years. Since it started, less than 5% of PEP graduates have returned to prison.

In the three years since Catherine started PEP, more than 300 inmates have walked in cap and gown ceremonies to graduate. More than 50% had previously committed violent crimes. These unique grads have been taught about entrepreneurship, ethics, family, racism, fatherhood, tithing, and topics important to developing their hearts so they can make it. Of all PEP graduates, 98% are employed within four weeks of release, and three grads made more than $100,000 in their first year after getting out.

More than 40 of these trained and motivated ex-convicts have gone on to start their own businesses, proving they can be entrepreneurial. The leather portfolio Catherine carries was made by an ex-prisoner who served 30 years for multiple murders and now creates purses and Bible covers. Other businesses have been started in power washing, computer services, landscaping, catering, and automotive repair.

Catherine recruited more than 800 CEOs and business leaders for active involvement in PEP. She started recruiting executives by sending letters to the CEOs of mid-size to billion-dollar companies, sharing what she had experienced. "I had a 10% hit rate on my first mailing campaign, which is pretty wild for a cold letter," she recalled. "Those CEOs were my first volunteers." Then she recruited from the political world as well. President George W. Bush sent PEP an unsolicited personal contribution, and Warren Buffet has written congratulatory letters for PEP graduates.

One CEO overheard an inmate share: "I'm an inmate, and my family lives 30 minutes away, and they never come to visit me. But these executives could be anywhere in the world, and they know all this stuff about business, and they come here to listen to my presentation." The prisoners know they matter, that they are worth something.

The current PEP class is creating and presenting comprehensive business pans to judging panels of business executives from across the nation. PEP has established partnerships with MBA programs and has a "fresh start" outlook, teaching principles of success: a servant-leader mentality, love, innovation, accountability, integrity, execution (a different kind than that of their past!), fun, excellence, and wise stewardship.

These one-time social cast-offs are also taught to give back. They personally know that the PEP re-entry scholarship costs about $750 per person. Astonishingly, more than two-thirds of PEP graduates voluntarily support the mission after release, having been taught the value of tithing and giving to others.

Catherine plans to enroll 200 to 250 or more Texas prison graduates a year and has visions of expanding to other states. There is no shortage of opportunities in her field of dreams. In reflecting on the significance of the past three years, she said: "I'm not superwoman. I'm a Lois Lane. I'm just a very normal person who decided to say 'Yes' to God." By setting inmates free through direction and coaching, and by monitoring their progress, new productive businessmen are unleashed.

Surrounded by hardened prisoners, Catherine uses her charm and passion to challenge inmates to succeed in life and become entrepreneurs, equipping them to create business plans to implement upon their release. It's not easy to gain the respect of hardened convicts, but Catherine Rohr has gained that, and more, by believing in them.

≋ *Ripples... by Alvin Hammons*

When I was very young, my Dad told me I was a loser. I got locked up in 1986 and was paroled in 1987. Unfortunately, I was no smarter than when I arrived. By the end of 1987, I was back with two concurrent sentences: life for attempted capital murder and 95 years for robbery.

I was granted parole in 2006 on the condition I complete a therapeutic treatment program at the Hamilton Unit. Although many people did not believe in me, Mom did. Mom found out about PEP before I was transferred and encouraged me to participate. I applied only at her urging. I completed the application honestly: I had 11 other felonies not prosecuted, 13 major cases, 18 minor cases, and was a high school drop out. I did well with mechanical skills, but "book learning" was not my thing. With all of that, I did not think Ms. Rohr would accept me into PEP—but she did.

I failed every test for the first several weeks of class. Why? Almost everyone knew I was a loser, and it was a lesson they had taught me well. I was failing, but determined to not disappoint Mom.

As class progressed, something else took hold. I met MBA students and business executives. Everyone talked to me with respect. My editor, Kami, told me I was doing well. Her encouragement stuck in my head. This lady did not know me, yet she believed in me. It was a good feeling. I started passing tests and feeling good about myself. It turned me around.

Either Ms. Rohr's insight or Mom's prayers paid off. On October 20, 2006, wearing a cap and gown, listening to Ms. Rohr tell the graduation audience all we had accomplished, experienced, and endured, I realized

I am no longer a loser. I am a winner. Along with three other guys, I received an award for the most improved participant.

Many of the business lessons may not have sunk in, but PEP gave me something much more valuable, something I have never had before. I found confidence in myself. I probably was not ready to return to the world when I arrived at Hamilton, but now I am. Honestly, I could not say that before I met Ms. Rohr and went through PEP. There is no doubt in my mind I will get out and succeed in life. I may never start my own business, but I know I will never come back to prison. That is true success.

P.S. — Alvin is a general manager for Bodart Recruiters. He picks up newly released ex-offenders from the bus stop and places them in housing that Bodart has secured. He also takes them to job interviews that have been lined up for them and then continues to take them to and from work. He manages the apartment complex where these men stay and must let them go if they are not conforming to the rules they agreed to abide by. The men he works with are not allowed to have vehicles, so he also finds himself taking them to do menial chores such as grocery shopping and general errands. He stays on call nearly 24 hours a day and works basically seven days a week. He really likes his job responsibilities and feels he is making a difference.

For More Information

In 2004, Catherine Rohr founded Prison Entrepreneurship Program in Texas to encourage inmates nearing release to be entrepreneurs and find success when they are mainstreamed back into society. Together with the support of almost 800 CEOs and community leaders, PEP has graduated more than 300 inmates in three years—with less than a 5% recidivism rate.

Break out of the mold and help set prisoners free from the cycle of crime. Contact:

Prison Entrepreneurship Program
PO Box 926274
Houston, Texas 77292-6274
Phone: (832) 767-0928
Website: www.pep.org

Joe Avila
Prison Fellowship

Making a U-Turn in Life

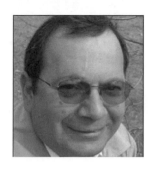

Life-changing events can take years, or a split second. For Joe Avila, 58, Prison Fellowship executive director for Central California and Nevada, it was the latter. In one horrifying moment in September 1992, screeching tires, shrieking brakes, smashing metal, and shattering of glass turned Joe's world upside down.

Joe was a family man living in Fresno, California with his wife, Mary, and daughters, Elizabeth and Grace. He made a good living as a site acquisition engineer with Nextel and McCaw Communications. His neighbors called Joe a "good family man," a man who helped his neighbors and the community, using his pickup truck to deliver supplies to the homeless shelter and games to church and school carnival fund-raisers.

But Joe Avila had a dark side. He was an alcoholic—a bad one with five drunk driving convictions, one of them a hit-and-run. Joe said his work was very competitive: "It was a lot of the world's stuff, and the heavy drinking went with it."

On September 18, 1992, while speeding drunkenly down a Fresno freeway, Joe Avila plowed his pickup truck into the rear of a car driven by a 17-year-old high school honor student and cheerleader. The girl died. A classmate in the car was severely injured. Joe fled the scene but was arrested a few hours later at his home.

Five days later, sitting with the chaplain in the Fresno County Jail, a deeply sobered and remorseful Joe became a Christian and asked God to redeem him from his life of sin and alcoholism. With his prior record and a manslaughter charge, Joe was looking at 12 years in prison. However, his attorneys wanted to fight the case. "Everybody does it, we'll get you off, just sign here," they told him.

When his trial date came up, the new Joe-in-Christ shocked his attorneys, ordering them to switch his plea to guilty. No plea-bargaining, no drawn out trial to drag his family and the victim's family through, just prepare for the maximum. The judge gave him 12 years. "You are an alcoholic," the judge said. "There is nothing this court can do to replace Miss Wall. There's going to be emptiness in the lives of her family and friends. Her death is an outrage."

Joe knew prison was never a delight, but he pledged to make it a learning experience. "I cherished every minute I spent behind bars because I was learning," Joe said. "People could see the change in me, and they can see the Christ-likeness in the redeemed. I got a chance to be involved with a lot of fellow prisoners and to actually lead people to the Lord."

Joe worked in the prison hospital and visited dying men in the hospice unit. "God gave me the privilege to represent His Son to the dying, the downhearted, and the diseased," he said. "I remembered how Jesus embraced the lepers, and I tried to be like Him in embracing men dying of AIDS or cancer. It was the greatest thing I have ever done."

Meanwhile, on the outside, his wife Mary waited. "We knew prison can tear a marriage up, especially with the phone calls and letters," Joe said. "She had to deal alone with the loss of her job, one that she had held for 20 years. The drive to the prison was more than two hours, but Mary and the children tried to make it once every three weeks; sometimes for the day, sometimes staying overnight for a second day. "I have a lot of honor and respect for those who visit prisoners," Joe said. "You have to go there, you have to wait in line, and often the environment isn't pleasant. They endure a lot."

Just before Joe's first Christmas behind bars, he heard about Prison Fellowship's Angel Tree and signed up his daughters. A volunteer at the Prison Fellowship Fresno office took the application and delivered the gifts to Elizabeth and Grace. When Joe heard their "Thank you, Daddy," over the phone, he said, "Thank you, God."

Then Joe discovered *Inside Journal*, the newspaper for prisoners published by Prison Fellowship. He began reading it and sharing it with his family. Even though Joe's daughters, ages 8 and 14, were receiving Angel Tree gifts, they used their limited family funds to buy gifts for other Angel Tree children. Grace, the youngest, wrote a letter to the imprisoned father of the girl she bought gifts for and eventually the letter was published in *Inside Journal*. Fellow prisoners read the letter in the paper and sought out Joe for his testimony.

Joe encouraged a greater Prison Fellowship presence at the facility and soon volunteers were conducting three or four seminars a year. "When you find someone who really cares about you and about your family, that has a profound effect on you," Joe said.

Joe came home from prison January 6, 1999, paroled after serving six and a half years. As he left the prison, he was handed $200 "gate money" in an envelope. Once he was in the van with his wife and sisters, he opened the envelope and saw the new $20 bills. "They gave me play money!" Joe exclaimed. He was unaware that the appearance of the $20 bill had been changed during his incarceration. That was just the beginning of Joe's adjustment to life on the outside.

"I went through a lot." Joe explained, "Sometimes I reflect back and think I'm still in prison. I would stand in the house and switch the lights on and off, on and off. It was just an awesome feeling to have control over them. In prison, you don't have control over the lights; you don't have control over anything."

Through his participation in Prison Fellowship programs at the prison, Joe had become acquainted with Austin Morgan, their Fresno Area Director. Austin was able to put Joe into a re-entry job at minimal wage, coordinating a Prison Fellowship fund-raising banquet in Fresno with Chuck Colson as speaker. Shortly before the banquet, Austin Morgan unexpectedly passed away, and the banquet became a celebration of his life. Within the year, Joe applied for the Prison Fellowship Area Director job and was hired in January 2000.

Joe's love of prisoners and his dedication to serving is evident. In his first Christmas with Prison Fellowship, he doubled the number of Angel Tree children served, reaching 13,021 boys and girls. He now covers the Fresno and Bakersfield, California, regions, plus southern Nevada, including Las Vegas. Nearly 50,000 prisoners are housed within his region, but he has already established programs in every facility and recruited volunteers to bring the positive messages of love to the prisoners.

Joe Avila has made a sharp U-turn in life since that day 14 years ago when his addiction to alcohol caused him to take an innocent life. However, even he and his wife, Mary, were unprepared for the miracles lying ahead. Just before Thanksgiving 2005, Joe and Mary, together with two mediators, met with Derek Wall, the brother of the girl Joe had killed. Derek was 15 at the time his sister died. He had heard Joe tell his story on a local radio program about drunk driving and had asked to meet him.

Face-to-face and eye-to-eye, they discussed how that tragic night had changed both their lives forever. Joe apologized and said he would continue to honor Amy Wall by sharing her story. Derek accepted the apology and gave Joe his keychain. It had Amy's photo on it and the inscription, "Someone drank and drove, and Amy died." Derek added the words "so that others might live" and gave it to Joe. With tears in their eyes, the two men shook hands and prayed.

Later, Derek wrote to Joe: "It is not by our own doing that our paths have crossed, nor is it by our doing that we are able to endure the tragedies we face. Not that I am pleased being without my sister, but in essence, she is not going alone. By her passing, she gave us a second chance in life—you, me, and all the lives we touch as a result of her. Every day, we all have choices to make, and I am grateful that others are making better choices because you have entered into their lives."

Joe Avila cannot reverse what happened that September evening on a Fresno highway. Nevertheless, he knows he is forgiven, not only by God but by the victim's family as well. As he uses his story to educate people about driving drunk, he prevents others from going through what he did.

That is his personal monument to Amy Wall.

For More Information

Founded in 1976 by Chuck Colson, *Prison Fellowship* offers love, hope, and direction to more than 2 million men and women incarcerated in America's prisons and jails. A total of 100,000 volunteers, across the nation and in 108 countries around the world, reach out to give hope to the hopeless. Colson has visited more than 600 prisons throughout the U.S. and the world. Some of the Prison Fellowship ministries include:

The InnerChange Freedom Initiative (IFI): A revolutionary, Christ-centered, Bible-based prison program that supports inmates and ex-cons through their spiritual and moral transformation. IFI conducts programs in Texas, Minnesota, Iowa, and Kansas. While the national recidivism (return to prison) rate is nearly 70%, in prisons with IFI/PF programs, it less than 10%.

Wilberforce Forum: Named for one of Colson's heroes, William Wilberforce—an 18th century British parliamentarian who stood against his party in a campaign to abolish the slave trade— the Wilberforce Forum teaches clear biblical views of Christian principles on current events and controversial issues affecting everyday life. It produces print magazines, web information and Colson's radio broadcast, *BreakPoint*, which is aired five times a week on 1,000 stations with an estimated nationwide audience of more than 1 million. Wilberforce Forum works to shape public policy on criminal justice reform, freedom of religion, and human rights.

Angel Tree: Founded in 1982 by Mary Kay Beard, a former prisoner and Prison Fellowship staff member, this ministry has given more than 7 million children of prisoners Christmas gifts in their incarcerated parents' names. Youth summer camping programs and mentoring opportunities also are offered.

Inside Journal: A newspaper circulated exclusively to inmates, *Inside Journal* offers Bible studies, guidance on getting through a prison sentence and on life after release, as well as advice on parenting and maintaining a marriage from behind bars.

Break out, reach out, and get involved by contacting:

Prison Fellowship

1856 Old Reston Avenue

Reston, Virginia 20190

Phone: (703) 478-0100; Fax: (703) 478-0452

Website: www.pfm.org

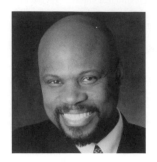

Wintley Phipps
U.S. Dream Academy

A Better Life for Children At Risk

"A child with a dream is a child with a future™"

—Motto of U.S. Dream Academy, Inc.

Wintley Phipps could rest easy on his laurels, if he wanted to. As a widely admired two-time Grammy-nominated singer and songwriter of Gospel and other religious music, his rich baritone has entertained presidents, celebrities, Mother Teresa, Nelson Mandela, and at the Vatican. He is also an ordained, spirit-filled minister and motivational speaker.

However, Wintley responded to a new challenge a decade ago when he served on the Board of Directors for Chuck Colson's Prison Fellowship. Colson, who was imprisoned in 1974–75 for his involvement in the Watergate scandal, insisted Wintley accompany him on prison visits, introducing the words and song of Phipps to prisoners across America.

Phipps had no idea he would come face-to-face with the reality of his own extended family's life: "I had just sung at a women's prison in Florida, when a very pregnant young woman asked me if my wife's name is Linda," he said. "When I confirmed it, she said with tears rolling down her face, 'she's my aunt.'"

Wintley would note that many brothers and sisters of his wife have either been in jail or incarcerated at some point in their lives. Then he saw a statistic that would change his life: "Between 60 and 70 percent of children of incarcerated parents may become inmates themselves. I had to do something about it."

That "something" became the U.S. Dream Academy, a nationally recognized after school program designed to empower young people to achieve their dreams. "It's a youth-focused program that speaks to the alarming cycle of inter-generational involvement in the criminal justice system," said Wintley. We want to lift the children of incarcerated parents and those failing in school out of this devastating cycle."

Eleven-year-old "J" is an example. Both of his parents have been in prison since he was seven. "J" lives with an aunt who said his school grades and behavior suffered until he enrolled at the U.S. Dream Academy program at his Houston elementary school.

"That changed everything," she said. "It sparked in him a new outlook on life and a desire to learn. He's smiling again; he's excited about going to class; he does his homework; he concentrates in school. Best of all, 'J's' grades are up, and this is all due to the U.S. Dream Academy."

Research suggests that as many as 80 percent of the people in prison and jails are high school dropouts. So the U.S. Dream Academy's program focuses on children in grades three through eight to try to reach them when they are academically most vulnerable. "I believe that I'm helping children to live out their own dreams," said Wintley, "to find their own voice and their own path in life."

The first U.S. Dream Academy opened in Southeast Washington, D.C. in early 2000. There are currently eleven learning centers around the country: two in Washington, D.C. and one each in Salt Lake City, Indianapolis, Los Angeles, Philadelphia, Baltimore, Orlando, Memphis, Houston, and East Orange, New Jersey.

More than 800 young people receive daily academic support through an online curriculum entitled Success Maker. Students also receive one-to-one mentoring from a caring adult.

"It's not the computers that will transform the lives of these kids," Wintley said. "The most important part of our program is the caring, loving adults who surround them. We know that the children we don't educate often become the adults we incarcerate. We want to demonstrate that with right tools and guidance, a child can achieve anything, regardless of how they got their start in life."

Wintley Phipps was born in Trinidad, West Indies and raised in Montreal, Quebec, Canada. He earned a bachelor's degree in theology and a Master of Divinity degree.

As a singer, he has performed for Presidents Jimmy Carter, Ronald Reagan, George H.W. Bush, Bill Clinton, and George W. Bush. He also sang at several National Prayer Breakfast events, the 1984 and 1988

Democratic National Conventions, Billy Graham Crusades, and for Pope John Paul II at the Vatican.

An ordained minister, humanitarian and visionary, Mr. Phipps inspires others to excellence and the realization of their life goals. "I was searching for effective ways to impact and transform the lives of young people who, without clear intervention, might find themselves following their parents to prison. The philosophy that guides my life is: '*There is a purpose and destiny for each life.*'"

For More Information

Founded by Grammy-nominated baritone Wintley Phipps in 2000, the U.S. Dream Academy is a national after-school program that empowers young people to fulfill their potential through skill-building, character-building, and dream-building activities. They focus their programs on at-risk boys and girls and children of parents in prison.

Sing out your dreams: break the cycle for children at risk and give them hope. Contact:

U.S. Dream Academy

10400 Little Petuxent Parkway, Suite 300

Columbia, Maryland 21044

Phone: (800) US DREAM

Website: www.usdreamacademy.org

Brittany Roach
Girl Scouts of the USA

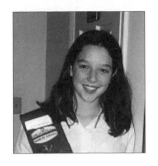

Youth: Courageous and Strong

It was supposed to be the trip of 12-year-old Brittany Roach's young life. Little did she know what challenges she and her family were about to face. For five consecutive months in 2001, the longtime Girl Scout had spent all her spare time collecting 3,000 pounds of toys, supplies, and other treats destined for poor orphaned children in Poland. She started the charitable project called "Collections for Kids" with her eyes set on earning Girl Scout's Highest Award for 11–14 year-olds—a Silver Award. While other girls her age in West Los Angeles were busy picking school outfits or shopping for CDs, Brittany coordinated drives that amassed loads of diapers, shoes, and even wheelchairs.

Poland wasn't Brittany's first choice. "My friend's dad owns an orphanage in China where we originally wanted to do something, but all the kids got adopted. We thought about Korea, but were told it would be too hard politically. Our neighbor suggested Poland because even though the Polish people don't have much, they will give you the shirts off their backs. So we went along with that idea." In the one-time Soviet occupied country, Brittany discovered that children and their families only dreamed of luxuries like a new toy or a mattress.

For five consecutive months in 2001, the longtime Girl Scout had spent all her spare time collecting 3,000 pounds of toys, supplies, and other treats destined for poor orphaned children in Poland.

Brittany's family crated a huge shipment destined for 350 children living in three Warsaw orphanages. Preparations had taken nearly a year, but from the outset the trip was an adventure of challenges and miracles. "I wrote first lady Laura Bush and asked if she could help us get our aid through customs," Brittany said. "Without hesitating, Mrs. Bush contacted the director of U.S. Customs, who then oversaw the shipment from Los Angeles to Warsaw." Northwest Airlines generously shipped the goods at no charge, and it looked like everything would go smoothly. The Polish kids were excited and sent Brittany letters and drew pictures.

Six weeks later, Brittany and her family set off for Eastern Europe to distribute the fruits of Brittany's labor in person. But upon arrival at London's Heathrow Airport, instead of boarding their connecting plane to Poland, they boarded an ambulance. Sometime during the flight from Los Angeles, Brittany's dad developed a blood clot that traveled to his brain. In the ambulance, he couldn't remember anyone's names, including his own. The stroke was so severe that her 50-year-old father, Guy, would have to re-learn basic skills like speaking and reading. Though Poland was no longer an option, Brittany never spoke of any disappointment at missing her "trip of a lifetime." Her priorities were focused solely on her dad.

As Brittany helped her father recuperate, using her small travel journal to patiently re-teach him numbers and colors, the 350 orphans still eagerly awaited the parties where the gifts were distributed. Polish Girl Guides, the Polish Girl Scout equivalent, handed out the toys and stuffed animals, toiletries and medical supplies. Back in London, the 100 stuffed animals Brittany had carried with her on the plane brought smiles to the children in the Pediatric Ward of the hospital where her father was being treated.

By the time the Roach family returned to California, letters, cards, and stories from the Polish orphans had begun trickling in. "There is this boy there named Krzysio," Brittany said. "He has cerebral palsy and can't walk. Krzysio received a wheelchair and crutches so he can play with his friends. We didn't get there ourselves, but I think we actually changed a lot of children's lives. It was really fun doing it, too."

Even before her ambitious project for Polish orphans, Brittany had organized clothing and shoe drives for children in Watts, a Los Angeles neighborhood scarred by decades of poverty and gang violence. Through her church youth group, she put together a van full of donations for 75 needy families.

Her impressive record of public service has not gone unnoticed. In a note sent directly from the White House, first lady Laura Bush thanked Brittany for her efforts: "You will never fully know the magnitude of the good you have done," Mrs. Bush wrote. "The ripples from your good works will keep spreading and spreading, touching lives in ways you could never have expected."

Brittany herself is a ripple, inspired by an organization started almost 100 years ago. Now **with 3.7 million members, Girl Scouts of the USA** has become famous for inspiring hundreds of thousands of young women and girls like Brittany to create service projects of their own. Through two world wars, the Great Depression and the Civil Rights Movement, Girl Scouting became a symbol of service for young girls throughout the nation.

Founded in 1912 by a Savannah, Georgia visionary named Juliette Gordon Low, the original troop had just 18 members. Juliette was so compelled by her dream of "giving the United States something for all the girls" that she sold her rare necklace of matched pearls to finance the initial operation. Think of that: Juliette's single, sacrificial gift of a pearl necklace changed the way of life for the youth of this nation for almost a hundred years—teaching character, service, morality and teamwork to girls who will become America's women. It was just Juliette's necklace plus her vision and energy that launched a movement which continues to grow almost 100 years later.

During World War I, Juliette's Girl Scouts labored in fields and hospitals growing vegetables and selling defense bonds. By 1920, the girls had their own uniform, handbook, constitution and by-laws, and in 1926, membership soared to 137,000. Ten years later, they licensed their first commercial baker to produce what became the inimitable **Girl Scout Cookie.**

Throughout the 20th century, this character-shaping organization often served unnoticed behind the backdrop of American history. During the Great Depression of the 1930s, Girl Scouts collected food and clothing and worked on community canning projects. In World War II, Scout troops served the home front collecting fat for soap, salvaging scrap metal and growing "Victory Gardens." Throughout its 95-year history, Girl Scouts has remained visionary, from its civil rights actions in the 1960s, to its "echo-action" projects of the 1980s and physical fitness programs of the 1990s.

For Brittany, Girl Scouting meant doing everything in her power—and beyond what she thought one person could do—to brighten the lives of people in her world. Her advice to others is simple: "Try and make a difference. My mom says we're God's vessels and that he works through us. It may just be a little thing, like when you're small and you bring cans of food for the homeless people. That helps. Just do anything you can. That's what the Girl Scouts taught me."

The Girl Scout Promise:

On my honor, I will try:
To serve God and my country,
To help people at all times,
And to live by the Girl Scout Law.

The Girl Scout Law:

I will do my best to be

honest and fair,
friendly and helpful,
considerate and caring,
courageous and strong, and
responsible for what I say and do,

and to

respect myself and others,
respect authority,
use resources wisely,
make the world a better place, and
be a sister to every Girl Scout.

Operation Thin Mint®

In 2002, a San Diego Girl Scout staffer had an idea with a flash of brilliance: send our deployed U.S. military troops "a taste of home and a note to show we care." Girl Scouts' San Diego Imperial Council entrepreneurial group started Operation Thin Mint® to ship celebrated Girl Scout cookies along with hand-written notes to deployed service

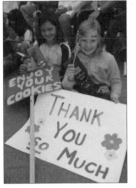

members. If prospective San Diegan cookie customers declined to buy cookies for themselves, they were given the irresistible opportunity to buy a box for U.S. troops. This win-win-win idea blossoms on all fronts: Girl Scouts benefit because cookie proceeds fund troop activities and the council's support services; our military personnel receive a special treat of a personalized gift; and San Diegans have an easy way to send their love to those serving our country far from home.

Thanks to APL, a generous company that provides free shipping, cookies sailed to Iraq, Afghanistan, Africa, Korea and other countries around the world. As the cookies and notes went out, the dough rolled in and the Girl Scout troops were blessed. By 2007, the Operation Thin Mint® program had sent well over one million boxes of cookies and countless notes for our military to enjoy.

With a highly motivated and adorable sales force of 2.7 million girls wearing vests and smiles, Girl Scouts make a mint with their Cookie Program. Girls annually sell about 200 million boxes at an average price of $3.50 per box. That girl-power adds up to $700 million of income each year to provide programs for girls, train adult volunteers, and provide financial assistance to ensure every girl has an opportunity to be a Girl Scout.

Through the Girl Scout Cookie Program, young women learn character, lifetime values and work ethic. The program not only raises money, it is a highly successful business and economic venture teaching teamwork, money management and goal setting.

San Diego Girl Scout troops are proud that Operation Thin Mint® turned into a profitable and meaningful program bringing smiles and a reminder of home to service members on the other side of the world.

Girl Scouting builds young ladies of courage, confidence, and character, who make the world a better place. It is the preeminent leadership development organization for girls.

Founded in 1912 by Juliette Low with just 18 members, Girl Scouts now consists of **3.7 million girls and adult members worldwide in 236,000 different troops** dedicated to service and building character. **Nearly one million adults volunteer with Girl Scouts of the USA** every year. Its sister organization, Girl Guides, is active in 90 countries around the world. Laura Bush is the national honorary president.

More than 50 million American women have been Girl Scouts and each knows the global impact rippling out. Each ripple starts at the hand of a little girl just like Brittany Roach.

March on, shore up the little troops, and support "girls growing strong." Contact:

Girl Scouts of the USA

420 Fifth Avenue

New York, New York 10018

Phone: (800) 478-7248

Website: www.girlscouts.org

Joe Heard

Representing: Kiwanis
International

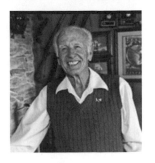

In Service to Children of the World

"I would like young people to realize they work against themselves when they say 'I can't.' If I could make it as a country boy from the farm, then anyone can make it."   —Joe Heard

Nearly 100 years ago, Joe Prance, a Detroit tailor, helped start a business and professional men's club to improve the lives of children in his area. For a name, he turned to an American Indian phrase, "Nunc Kee-wan-is," which means "We have a good time; we make a big noise." Six months later, the 200 members dropped the first word, and "Kiwanis" was off and running. Their first major service project was to adopt a young ward. They changed his name to Henry Kiwanis.

Today, that organization is known as Kiwanis International, and it has more than 8,000 Kiwanis clubs in 96 countries, with a membership of more than 260,000. Another 320,000 young people participate in 7,000 Kiwanis youth clubs: "K-Kids" for elementary-age children, "Key Club" for high school students, and "Circle K" for collegians. Living out their motto, "Serving the Children of the World," Kiwanis members work to develop future generations of leaders. Every day, they revitalize neighborhoods, organize youth sports programs, tutor, build playgrounds, children's hospitals, and regional homeless shelters, and perform countless other projects that help children and communities.

How can we best relate the vast and remarkable achievements of this large and active organization that has been helping children worldwide for nearly a century? Let's zoom in on one Kiwanis member as an example.

Joe Heard has been a driving force behind 18 Kiwanis clubs around San Diego, California, and their joint effort to help homeless children in Romania. The son of an Alabama sharecropper, Joe grew up with six brothers and a sister in the rough years between the Depression and World War II. With virtually no education, he worked in farm fields. At age 18, he enlisted with the U.S. Marines, where he spent 30 years on an unusual military career path. "Thank God I was selected to attend the University of Southern California under a special Navy program where I was educated and majored in cinema," Joe said. "I received a field commission and served as the Marine Corps' photographic officer. For 13 years, part of my responsibility was to provide television and motion picture coverage for the President of the United States of America."

On retiring from the military in 1978, Joe moved to Escondido, near San Diego, and ran a construction company. Along the way, he joined the Escondido Kiwanis club, where he became both president of the local club and coordinator for the 18 Kiwanis clubs in San Diego's North County.

In the year 2000, the Romanian transition training team became a reality and was undertaken by Joe's Kiwanis Division. Joe accompanied his friends Jim Sorrels and Pete Zindler to Romania in 2003, where they ministered to orphans through Heart 2 Heart, a nonprofit organization founded by Sorrels. Joe's heart broke when he saw the plight of the estimated 200,000 orphans and abandoned children living on the streets and in the sewers. When a frail little boy walked over to Joe and tugged at his pants leg, Joe saw hunger and hopelessness in the boy's sad eyes. "He was skinny as a rail. Dogs were treated better than these kids," Joe said.

The majority of Romanian children were abandoned by their parents under the Ceausescu Communist regime. The dictator had outlawed birth control and required every woman of childbearing age to have five children or be heavily taxed. Couples who had children they didn't want or couldn't afford were allowed to abandon them at the local hospital—no questions asked. Poverty and the discarding of children have continued there since the fall of communism in 1989.

When Joe returned to San Diego, he could not forget the haunting eyes of the boy who had tugged at his pants. When he tried to make a presentation to his Kiwanis club, "I stood up and I didn't get three words out of my mouth when I busted up crying, thinking of those kids," Joe recalled. That day, his testimony about the plight of Romania's children touched the hearts of his fellow Kiwanis members. Joe became a man on a mission, bringing all 18 North County Kiwanis clubs into partnership with Heart 2 Heart for a Romanian foster home sponsorship program.

Through their joint efforts, the number of homeless children in Romania dropped dramatically.

But Joe wasn't even close to finished. He saw that Romanian children who were not placed in foster homes were forced to move out of the orphanage at age 18. Lacking family support and life skills, the teens quickly sank into an empty, desperate life on the streets. Joe, his Kiwanis team, and Heart 2 Heart raised money to build transition homes for boys and opened a boy's training center in 2003.

Girls in Romanian orphanages, like the boys, were pushed onto the street at age 18 with no money or education. Most of them fell immediately into prostitution. The orphanage director asked if a home and transition program could be started to allow the girls to get some education. The girls' house opened a year after the boys'.

Both programs provide a temporary home for a year or more. The boys learn auto mechanics, woodworking, bicycle repair, and baking. When Joe arranged for a welding machine, local Romanian companies gave spare steel. The boys used their new welding skill to produce a handsome wrought iron fence for the center. When nearby residents saw their work, they quickly placed paid orders for fences of their own. A cheese factory project is underway, as well as greenhouses where the boys can raise produce to sell.

The girls also learn life skills and job training, especially in sewing, office work, and hairstyling. Many of the girls find permanent employment before leaving the center. Students at both centers learn computer skills through a large donation of computers and software from Dell, arranged by Joe and his Kiwanis teammates. "It has changed their lives!" Joe exclaims. "Now the girls and boys in our program have their own school system, and on weekends they have an opportunity to socialize in park-like settings."

On another Romanian trip, Joe's Kiwanis group met with the mayor of a town. "When we walked in to their facility, the mayor said 'We need books so we can learn about America.' We gladly sent pallets of books and computers," Joe said. "And since bicycles are the main transportation for young people, we just sent 150 bicycles, thanks to the police departments of San Diego and Escondido. We also sent bicycles in parts and pieces so our boys can learn how to repair the bikes and take care of them."

Joe and Kiwanis colleague Dave Imper work nearly full time, backstopping Heart 2 Heart in its service to the children of Romania. Their next project: a 144-bed training center to be built on 10 acres of land donated by the government. Joe and Dave recently were named finalists for the 2008 Kiwanis World Service Medal.

Joe Heard may be in his 70s now, but he is young at heart and passionate about the needs of children, both in the United States and Romania. He has no plans for retiring from his mission. Like Kiwanis' founder, Joe Prance, Joe Heard and all Kiwanis members take pride in their commitment to serve the world's children.

≋ *Ripples...*

Kiwanis ripples and a few examples of key miracle-makers in action:

IDD Initiative ≈ All children deserve the best possible start in life. Yet every day babies around the world are born at risk of iodine deficiency disorder (IDD), which not only causes goiter, but also may result in irreversible brain damage in a fetus or infant and cause retarded psychomotor development in children. Iodine deficiency is the most common cause of preventable mental retardation.

In 1994, Kiwanis launched its first World-Wide Service Project in partnership with the United Nations Children's Fund (UNICEF) to eliminate IDD. The campaign has raised nearly $100 million, which it has since invested in 95 developing countries.

The entire Kiwanis family worked together to help eliminate the problem of IDD by supporting salt iodization, testing and monitoring, community outreach, and education. The percentage of iodized salt worldwide has been raised from 30% to 70%, and UNICEF estimates more than 80 million children in the developing world will be born free of iodine deficiency disorder in 2007.

Heralded by UNICEF as one of the greatest public health triumphs of the 20th century, members of the Kiwanis family can take great pride in their accomplishments. Today about 70% of people in the developing world have access to iodized salt. Through the Kiwanis family's dedication and hard work, not only in raising money but also in raising awareness of the problem and motivating governments and industry to act, millions of children have been protected against the invisible but devastating effects of iodine deficiency.

Camp Beyond the Scars ≈ When he was nine years old, Corey Repucci was trapped in his bedroom as a fire raced through his house. He suffered third-degree burns over 48% of his body. Now, thanks to Kiwanis, Corey and 70 other children with severe scars can again attend summer camp—Camp Beyond the Scars in San Diego. They spend eight days swimming, mountain biking, doing crafts, playing games, and healing—both physically and emotionally. "When I first started coming here, I was real self-conscious about my burns," Corey said. "I started coming to the camp to go through the support system." After seven years of summer camps, 17-year-old Corey is a counselor-in-training, hoping to encourage younger burn victims in need.

The Miracle League Field ≈ Travel to Montgomery, Alabama, and you can visit a unique field of dreams where children with autism and disabilities can play baseball and organized sports, thanks to Kiwanis members. Jimmy Hook is a nine-year-old autistic cherub who excitedly signed up the first day the program opened. He had never been able to play organized sports with other kids. "Little League or Dixie Youth Leagues are just not set up for someone like me," Jimmy said.

Donning a shirt and a hat, Jimmy ran onto the field and took a batter's stance at home plate. "When I hit the ball, Dad carried me to first base, and then I ran with him to second, and third, and HOME!" Jimmy exclaims. "That was enough for me that first day. You see, I have problems in crowds sometimes, and I just have to get away from all the people and noise." Jimmy went back week after week, however, and practiced at home all winter. Now he plays on his own. Jimmy loves sliding into all the bases and can hit the ball all the way to the fence. And he is not alone. Teammates play ball on miracle fields around the country—all supported by Kiwanis members who ache to serve children like Jimmy.

Reading is Fundamental ≈ Select books. Order books. Sort books. Find a better way to sort books. Deliver books. Read books. Write books. Keith Baldwin and his Copper County Houghton (Michigan) Kiwanis chapter coordinate "Reading is Fundamental" projects three times every year, collecting thousands of books and conducting reading motivation activities for third-graders in nine school districts across an 800-mile rural area. Keith, a United States Army veteran and Michigan Tech University physics professor emeritus, uses his ingenuity and the help of volunteers from Michigan Tech's Circle K club and area Key Clubs to raise funds, deliver books, and conduct reading parties. Recently, they sponsored a contest for third-graders in which each class composed a story that started with the line, "Once upon a time, there was a magical book that hopped off the shelf into the hands of ...." Keith has been heading this program for 25 years, and he continually runs into adults who have fond memories of participating in the program as a child.

Inner City Kiwanis ≈ Young, energetic Erica Hauck had been taking leftover food from her company's lunches and giving it to homeless people on Skid Row a block from her downtown office. Her friend Camille invited the marketing and business development executive to join Kiwanis in 2001. After joining, Camille and Erica went with the Kiwanis Club to read to children in a downtown homeless shelter. A little boy named Willy latched on to her. "He wanted to hold my hand, to sit on my lap," Erica recalled. "He wanted me to read to him. He just needed attention so badly."

When Erica became Kiwanis lieutenant governor, she decided to revitalize an almost defunct group of downtown Los Angeles clubs called Division I. This area has now opened four clubs including one in Crenshaw in the South Central area and one in Mid Wilshire. She passionately desires to tap into the next generation of Kiwanis. "What drives my passion is that there are a lot of little Willies running around LA," Erica said. "If Division I went away, there would be fewer chances for these kids' lives to be touched. It's our duty."

All Dolled Up ≈ When it comes to getting a positive return on an investment of time, the Kiwanis Club of Bristol, Tennessee, has the market all sewn up. When the club decided to participate in a district-wide doll project, members cut out, stitched, stuffed, and sewed some 1,024 dolls—more than double their original goal of 500. The dolls are distributed among hospitals and child advocacy centers in the area, and are used by doctors as a child-friendly way of explaining illnesses or upcoming surgical procedures to children. The child can draw facial features on the dolls and dress them up, and even have visitors sign them as a reminder of the time they were in the hospital.

Pediatric Trauma Institute ≈ In Boston, the New England Kiwanis District supports the Kiwanis Pediatric Trauma Institute at the Tufts-New England Medical Center. For more than 30 years, this Kiwanis partnership has delivered ongoing support to provide much-needed trauma care for children throughout New England. Kiwanis has raised more than $7 million for this effort—and they are not alone. Chapters throughout the world support children's hospitals in a myriad of ways.

Aktion Clubs Act for the Disabled ≈ Kiwanians who live with disabilities know their limitations do not make them any less a member of the Kiwanis family. They do whatever they can to help their communities, and their service is a testament to the adage, "While no one can do everything, everyone can do something."

Kelley Kaplan, charter president of the Aktion Club of Eastern Carolina in Greenville, North Carolina, wanted to volunteer as a youth, but doors closed because she was labeled "retarded." When the Aktion Club opened in her area, Kelley's world expanded. "Finally, I am able to give back to the community that has given so much to me," she shares. She and her club made and auctioned artistic hearts, raising $4,700. When Kelley met a single mother whose son, Jackson, had severe cerebral palsy, she was proud to write a check for almost $400 on behalf of their club to buy Jackson a special wheelchair.

Whether participating in the Cancer Survivor Walk, rolling balls in a bowl-a-thon, marching in a Christmas parade, singing carols at a retirement home, or ringing the bells for the Salvation Army, Kelley's Aktion Club puts smiles on faces and makes a difference for people in need. Go Kelley! Go Aktion members all over the country and the world! You rock!

The Kiwanis Family House ≈ Gary Christensen becomes emotional and his heart pounds when he visits the families of sick children housed at the 19,500 square foot, 32-bedroom Kiwanis Family House in Sacramento, California. Gary and fellow Kiwanis members completed construction of the house in July 2006. Located by a Children's Miracle Network hospital, University of California Davis Medical Center, the beautiful facility is home to families in crisis who otherwise would sleep in a hospital waiting room or in their cars, anxious to be near a child being treated for a serious illness or injury.

Gary's passion goes back to the early 1980s, when he and Sacramento Kiwanians became aware that some families from outside the area could not afford temporary housing while their children were in medical crisis. The local Kiwanis club initially purchased, assembled, and renovated five modular buildings on a site donated by the UC Davis Medical

Center. They opened their doors in 1984, providing seven bedrooms, a community kitchen, and shower facilities for the families.

Their dream grew as they witnessed the need of families who came to this hub of medical hope for help. "We were often turning away 10 families a day, due to lack of space," Gary recalled. With an average stay of two weeks, this original house served 11,000 families. In 2000, Gary helped lead a six-year Kiwanis campaign to raise $4.5 million to construct a new facility, equipped with four kitchens, a laundry room, a children's game room, an outdoor playground, a conference room, and seven RV spaces. Each bedroom has a private bath, and the $15 per night fee is waived for the economically disadvantaged through the Mooretown Rancheria Club's "Sponsor A Family Program."

The award-winning Kiwanis Family House is an on-going project for Sacramento clubs that log nearly 10,000 volunteer hours every year, as well as raise money needed for its support. Offering hands-on assistance to financially needy families in crisis is a prime example of the heart, passion, and commitment of passionaries like Gary and the Sacramento Kiwanians.

Rose Parade Float Volunteers ≈ Kiwanis members do good *for* children and have productive fun *with* children as well. One prime example is how members build a float to deliver the Kiwanis message in the Pasadena Tournament of Roses Parade on New Years Day. Since 1986, 400 million people every year enjoy the spectacular float—but there is much more to this story.

In 1995, Kiwanis passionary Margo Dutton coordinated volunteers to decorate the Kiwanis float with roses and flowers. So many excellent high school student volunteers signed up that she decided to see if Kiwanis members could help decorate other floats as well. Thirteen years later, Margo coordinates Kiwanis volunteers who decorate one-fourth of all Rose Parade floats. Of the 7,000 volunteers, about 95% are high school Key Club members, drawing from Southern California, Nevada, and Oregon, with some even flying in from the East Coast.

Margo has watched young volunteer leaders blossom into Key Club governors and lieutenant governors after involving groups from their school in fun, productive, safe New Year's Eve activities. "On the surface, it may seem like putting pretty flowers on a float, but it is so much more," Margo said. "Leaders of tomorrow are stretching their wings on many fronts with the parade float activities." Margo's volunteers sow the seeds of leadership and inspire the buds and blooms of tomorrow's pioneers.

Find out more at about germinating volunteer opportunities at www.kiwanisrosefloat.com.

For More Information

The Kiwanis Family is a worldwide club of community leader volunteers dedicated to changing the world, one child and one community at a time. Kiwanis offers an opportunity for service and fun while improving the community, the nation, and the world, creating heart-shared friendships that are sincere and lasting.

Since its founding in 1915, Kiwanis and its Service Leadership Programs boast a membership of more than 600,000 men, women, and youth in nearly 16,000 clubs in more than 96 countries and geographic areas. Kiwanians volunteer more than 21 million hours and invest more than $113 million in their communities around the world.

Kiwanis continues its service emphasis of "Young Children: Priority One," which focuses on the special needs of children from prenatal development to age five. It focuses on the needs of children in pediatric trauma, safety, childcare, early development, infant, health, nutrition, and parenting skills. In a typical year, "Young Children: Priority One" service projects involve more than $14 million and 1 million volunteer hours. In 1994, Kiwanis launched its first World-Wide Service Project (WSP), a $75-million campaign in partnership with UNICEF to eliminate iodine deficiency disorders. IDD projects have been funded in 95 nations. Kiwanis International Foundation has raised nearly $100 million to eliminate IDD worldwide.

Kiwanis International is the only service organization building leaders at every level—from the youngest Kiwanis Kids through several youth and adult programs, including:

♥ CKI (Circle Kiwanis International): on 550 college and university campuses

- ♥ Key Leaders: a new leadership experience for exceptional leaders from 8th to 12th grades
- ♥ Key Club: 245,000 high school service leaders working on a variety of social causes
- ♥ Builder's Club: 40,000 middle and junior high students implementing service-learning principles
- ♥ K-Kids: service clubs for elementary students, teaching the value of helping others
- ♥ Terrific Kids recognizes character with prizes for: "Thoughtful, Enthusiastic, Respectful, Responsible, Inclusive, Friendly, Inquisitive, Capable kids
- ♥ BUG – Bringing Up Grades: recognizes students who improve their grades
- ♥ AKTION: 200 clubs allowing adults with disabilities to serve with initiative and leadership skills

In high schools and colleges, Key Club and Circle K are the largest service organizations of their kind in the world today. Every Kiwanis meeting engenders fun, service, and camaraderie.

Care best for children, for community, for yourself, with a local Kiwanis group. Contact:

Kiwanis International: check out a club close by where you live OR connect with:

3636 Woodview Trace

Indianapolis, Indiana 46268

Phone: (800) KIWANIS

Website: www.kiwanis.org

Points of Light & HandsOn Network

The following two parallel profiles focus on remarkable women connected by a passion to serve in two totally different ways—yet they end up being connected to the same organization, Points of Light Institute & HandsOn Network. Enjoy meeting Michelle and Debbie, who are shining points of light!

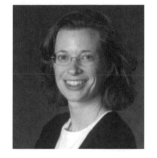

Michelle Nunn
CEO, *Points of Light Institute*
Co-Founder, *HandsOn Network*

An Amazing Vision

"I am a passionate believer that everyone has the possibility to take action that changes the world. Our communities and our democracy depend on that."

—Michelle Nunn

Michelle Nunn enthusiastically believes in facilitating opportunities for people to work together. By partnering with volunteer organizations and productively channeling the energy of givers, she is actively pursuing her vision of growing from 61 million Americans who presently volunteer to 100 million in the next few years.

She started in 1989 with HandsOn Atlanta, where she was its co-founder and first staff member. Michelle used her Southern charm and steel grit to help grow the nonprofit organization into 37,000 local volunteers, building community and meeting critical needs in schools, parks, senior homes, food banks, pet shelters, and low-income neighborhoods. From Atlanta, Michelle's idea spread to New York, Washington, D.C., and Chicago. Within 15 years, it became a national movement.

In 2007, HandsOn Network merged with the Points of Light Foundation (POLF) creating the world's largest global volunteer network. The new organization, Points of Light Institute, oversees a portfolio of business units—including HandsOn Network and MissionFish. HandsOn Network serves more than 80% of the American population and 12 international communities. The vast majority of Points of Light Institute's work and activity happens through 380 HandsOn Network Action Centers and its expanded network of hundreds of nonprofit, community, faith-based, government, and corporate organizations.

So what is HandsOn Network?

"We ensure that there are volunteer and community participation opportunities for people throughout the country and increasingly, around the world," Michelle said. "We engage individuals, corporations, nonprofits and government institutions to incubate, develop and mobilize collaborative citizen leadership—creating innovative, actionable solutions that can be replicated anywhere in the world. When HandsOn connects passion and action, transformation is possible. People can be transformers in their communities unleashing energy that creates the change we wish to see in the world."

One example was the disaster relief program in New Orleans, Louisiana, and Biloxi, Mississippi, following hurricanes Katrina and Rita. HandsOn activated more than 7,000 volunteers for daily revitalization projects, including school renovations and other community development programs.

"When HandsOn connects passion and action, transformation is possible. People can be transformers in their communities unleashing energy that creates the change we wish to see in the world."

In partnership with the Corporation for National and Community Service, HandsOn Network provides opportunities for more than 2 million Americans of all ages and backgrounds to serve through Senior Corps, Retired Senior Volunteer Program (RSVP), Learn and Serve America, and AmeriCorps. The AmeriCorps program alone mobilizes more than 100,000 youth volunteers nationwide. AmeriCorps Alums, a trained change-force more than 400,000 strong, has its headquarters at HandsOn Network.

Another key strategy of the organization, the HandsOn Network Corporate Council, has worked as a unified force to lead and inspire Corporate America toward increased civic impact. Founded in partnership with Bob Nardelli and The Home Depot, the Council has grown to include more than 60 CEOs and civic leaders representing some of the nation's largest and most successful Fortune 500 companies. With the merger, the Points of Light Foundation brought new talent and resources to the Council with the integration of the POLF National Council on Workplace Volunteerism (NCWV). The two Councils have come together, leveraging the strength and experience of their respective histories to create a clear vision and strategy for the future.

Of the thousands of projects that now fall within her organization, Michelle has a few favorites. One is the Discovery Program, started by Atlanta volunteer Richard Goldsmith. Richard was a plumbing executive who wanted to make a difference in the lives of young people. He wrote a newspaper article about a low-performing school, which got him an appointment with the school's principal—who challenged Richard to bring in some caring adults to help the school improve. The children needed mentoring and tutoring beyond school hours, the principal explained. The following Saturday, Richard and 25 friends showed up to tutor. They were greeted by hundreds of children, who wanted to start "Saturday School."

That was 17 years ago. The program has since expanded to dozens of Atlanta-area schools, but Richard still leads the program at that same school, where he is called "Mr. HandsOn." Former students come back in on Saturdays to mentor a new generation of children. While the Discovery Program has made a tangible difference in the lives of so many children, it has also changed Richard's life—he met his wife, another volunteer, while serving at the school.

Another favorite of Michelle's is Team Works, which began with the idea that many people would like to volunteer in various areas but don't know where to start. Team Works became a virtual "Volunteer 101" course where people were presented with the opportunity to learn about different issues. Groups that study together become teams that choose one area to focus on together.

Team Works has since become a much broader program called Citizen Academy, which enables people to engage in direct service, and also learn about various issues, such as how their school boards work. That in turn prompts volunteers to take a more active role, such as running for the school board. Michelle said, "It's about using the platform of direct service to show how people can make change and join in from a civic perspective."

It was through her family that Michelle came to public service. "I grew up in a home where service was always considered a part of our lives," she said. "It was an idea I was introduced to early on, and the values were critical motivators when I left college to return to Atlanta."

One of Michelle's grandfathers was a mayor. Her father is Sam Nunn, the former U.S. Senator from Georgia. Former Georgia Congressman Carl Vinson also is part of her family tree. "When one is introduced to public service at an early age, they likely will continue it," Michelle notes. "That was my experience, and I found satisfaction and meaning in it. I was able to be a mentor in high school, so it was a big shaper of my worldview, my life, and my perspectives."

Michelle wants to see the merged Points of Light & HandsOn Network become a powerful infrastructure in which everyone can realize their ability to change the world. "I think people want to be a part of something larger than themselves and that is just a common human impulse," she said. "People see all around them that they can truly make a difference, through their votes, their consumer choices, or through giving their time and money."

As a change-agent, Michelle is excited about transformational technologies that can bring people together. "We want to help everyone discover the power to make a difference and to be called on," she explained. "People want to do something and to be part of something bigger than themselves. That's where we come in."

Michelle currently serves on the President's Council on Service and Civic Participation and has been named by the *Non-Profit Times* as one of the "Power and Influence Top 50." Managing the newly merged organization is much more than a full-time job; it is a commitment to a lifestyle of service. Add in a family—husband Ron Martin, and two children—and you discover someone with seemingly unlimited energy. That's Michelle, a force of nature, harnessing people-power, building communities, witnessing miracles—and she's got big dreams for our future.

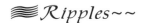

Christopher Calabia. After relocating to New York City, Chris found his new job in financial regulation exciting but demanding. "I set goals to explore New York and make more friends beyond the office," Chris said of his first months. "Having volunteered since high school, I thought that getting involved in the community again might do good for both myself and others at the same time."

Through a family friend, Chris learned about a small agency that served formerly homeless adults. He began volunteering there but found it taxing, as volunteers were expected to serve every Saturday from nine to five and some weekdays if possible. "I was in my mid-twenties, had just completed the rigors of graduate study, and was admittedly not ready to give up so many Saturdays," Chris explained.

Then a colleague told him about New York Cares. At the time, it was a relatively new agency with a novel approach that allows volunteers to choose from a wide range of projects and requires no long-term commitments. Chris was initially dubious about the program's business model but liked its flexibility and varied opportunities.

Soon he was volunteering far more than he anticipated, helping teams paint classrooms and community centers, clean and garden in public parks, all while becoming acquainted with neighborhoods and other civic-minded New Yorkers across the city. Eventually he chaired several New York Cares committees that planned large-scale service projects and spent almost eight years organizing monthly recreational and educational field trips for children living in family shelters in Harlem.

Today, Chris is a vice president at the financial regulatory agency. In the almost fourteen years since he first got involved, New York Cares has grown to nearly 36,000 volunteers and is an Action Center within the HandsOn Network. Some volunteer only occasionally, others quite frequently, but together they make a difference in the lives of almost 400,000 New Yorkers in need. Chris found that volunteering changed his life, too. On one stormy "New York Cares Day" devoted to serving public schools, Chris met a rain-drenched volunteer who later became his wife.

Jersey Cares based in Newark, New Jersey connects thousands of local volunteers to innovative programs—including the Jersey Cares Coat Drive which collected and distributed more than 30,000 coats to those in need in 2007. Their corporate service program has engaged volunteers in rock climbing wall installation projects, bicycle building sessions, financial literacy and job readiness workshops, beach clean-ups, and school makeovers. Way to go, Jersey!

The Volunteer Connection of Northwest Ohio brings people and assets together to meet social problems head-on. Their programs include Healing Hearts which is a support group for parents who have lost a child and Hunger Awareness Day which is a community food drive supplying tons of items to local food pantries each year. Recently, they partnered with the government to provide relief to victims of devastating floods.By bringing together her family and volunteers, they personally assisted an 84-year-old woman by gutting, cleaning and rebuilding her house in four months. She was able to return to her home on Christmas Eve, complete with a new, beautifully decorated Christmas tree. They are ready to be first-responders, serving their community needs on a daily basis. Fight on, Northwest Ohio!

Make a Difference (Phoenix, Arizona) has galvanized volunteers for the past 15 years to revitalize neighborhoods, provide meals to the homeless, support seniors in need, and create effective community partnerships. They engage more than 14,000 people a year, hosting between 40 and 50 volunteer projects each month, and contribute more than 50,000 hours of service to their community annually. Their outreaches include mentoring and tutoring programs such as Bookwork Buddies, which brings caring adults into Central Phoenix classrooms to assist teachers in helping fourth graders with reading and writing skills. They are the lead volunteer group coordinating emergency relief preparedness, as well as managing a serve-a-thon for Schools where 3,000 volunteers donate one day each year to make the Arizona Valley's schools a better place to learn. You rock, Phoenix volunteers!

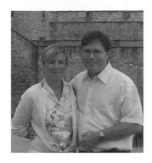

Debbie Spaide
Kids Care Clubs

The Power of Small Hands

When Debbie Spaide took her five young children to the home of an elderly woman whose yard needed work, she never dreamed it would be the beginning of a nationwide charity group for kids.

She and her husband, Jim, with the help of a social worker, organized that day trip in 1988 to keep her Connecticut family from becoming spoiled by the conveniences of a nice home, closets filled with clothes, and a pantry of hearty food. The couple wanted their kids to grow up more concerned about the value of their character than the price of their clothes. So they put rakes in their children's hands—all were less than 13 years old—and they all went to work on the yard.

A funny thing happened that day as the family raked and planted and clipped. Nobody complained. Nobody said they'd rather be home watching videos or at the mall with friends. Instead, other children began showing up, gloves and rakes in hand.

One of their older children had told some friends about the excursion, and word spread through the local middle school that the family was planning to help out again in the community. Fifteen pre-teens showed up that day, begging to help with the neglected yard. They worked alongside the Spaide family until everyone had blistered hands and earth-stained knees. On that day, all the common preconceptions of suburban children—that they were spoiled, self-involved youngsters too lazy to serve in their communities—blew away with the yard clippings. Debbie realized these kids weren't selfish or apathetic. They were dying to help, but in the age of swimming lessons and suburbia, many hadn't been given the chance.

Unlike Jim and Debbie's childhoods, this new generation of youngsters lived in a transient culture where they didn't know their neighbors. They didn't know what it was like to hop down the block to help their grandmother or take care of family friends with new babies. These kids were thirsty for some kind of affirmation. "Our children didn't have the same opportunity as we did growing up to serve others, to help people, to feel like they have something important to contribute," Debbie said. "So that's how it started."

What started as a family outing became the first project for what would soon be named the Kids Care Clubs. In the next few months, the couple began holding kids' meetings in their kitchen, trying to find community service work for children and young teens. They helped mow lawns, paint homes, and bag lunches for soup kitchens.

Word of the group and its good deeds spread like wildfire. In a few weeks, the group grew to 50 students, and within a year Debbie Spaide began getting calls from schools, churches, synagogues and mosques, all looking to start their own Kids Care Clubs. Seventeen years after the Spaide's first project, the notion that kids can make a difference has become an international phenomenon.

Today, there are more than .75,000 kids in 1,400 registered Kids Care Clubs in the United States, Canada, Europe, Africa, and Asia. Last year, Kids Care Clubs contributed millions of dollars in gifts and service through hands-on projects, including Team Up for Kids in Foster Care, Winter Wear Share, Animal Friends, Summer Shelter Helpers, Honoring Dr. Martin Luther King Jr., Earth Day Everyday, Operation Kids Care: Words for the Wounded, Holiday Hope Chests, and Eat Wise—Exercise!™ Through Kids Care Club projects, members have helped the elderly, hungry, homeless, disabled, sick, and victims of disaster.

One of those helped was 12-year-old Chris, a Massachusetts boy who awoke from a coma to find a Kids Care Club goody bag next to his hospital bed. Chris, who was suffering from back surgery complications, was so touched by the gift that he rallied his friends to help make placemats for elderly people at a neighborhood nursing home. Helping others gave Chris the joy and confidence to overcome his own physical and emotional wounds. "His mother said it was the most healing thing for him—to be able to be a leader, to have something important to give," Debbie recalled.

The success of Kids Care inspired Debbie Spaide to create the FamilyCares Network, a similar organization that helps families—not just kids—find opportunities to serve their communities. Raising money to sustain the two groups became a full-time job, and Jim and Debbie realized they could no longer manage them. So they turned the clubs over to the Points of Light Foundation, a government-funded organization also dedicated to getting children, from toddlers to teens, involved in service. In 2007, Points of Light merged and became Points of Light & HandsOn Network.

"Looking back," Debbie said, "forming the Kids Care Clubs was one of the biggest challenges of our family life." As they learned that first crisp morning in Connecticut, finding children and teens willing to serve their communities was the easy part. But finding organizations that would accept help from youngsters—and convincing the social service sector that even the smallest child has something to contribute—took perseverance and passion.

"Kids Care crosses all economic boundaries, and we even started clubs in homeless shelters. The need to contribute is within every child. Nobody at that time was interested in having kids of that age help. No, thank you! But little by little, the kids really won everybody over," Debbie said. "We had organizations calling us and saying, 'Here's what we need. Do you think the kids can help?'"

So how did the Spaides go from being a couple of do-gooders begging for kids' service opportunities to creating hundreds of service clubs? Slow, steady progress and taking joy in the everyday battles. "Most people who are making things happen are not superheroes. They're putting one foot in front of the other," Debbie continued. "Don't think about the final result or the big job, just take one step at a time." She urges others not to "get caught up in the reasons you can't do something—just do it and move forward. Listen for what's genuine. Whatever that genuine voice within us is telling us to do, from doing the dishes to managing a Fortune 500 company, it matters.

"From the littlest act to the largest act...every single thing we do matters to someone, somehow, somewhere. It could matter more than we will ever know."

In 1989, Michelle Nunn founded a volunteer organization called HandsOn Atlanta, a nonprofit that helps individuals, families, corporate, and community groups find flexible volunteer opportunities at over 400 service organizations and schools. HandsOn Atlanta quickly blossomed into a group of affiliates based on the same model of service. It grew to include 73 affiliate organizations across the country and around the globe.

In August 2007, the Points of Light Foundation formed by President George H. W. Bush in 1990, merged with HandsOn Network, creating the largest volunteer organization in the country. Under the leadership of CEO Michelle Nunn, Points of Light Institute oversees a portfolio of business units to empower Americans and help coordinate and acknowledge the millions of volunteers who work through a host of inspirational programs under its umbrella. Its groups include HandsOn Network, 1-800-VOLUNTEER.org, 50+ Volunteering Initiative, AmeriCorps, Promise Fellows Program, Disaster Preparedness & Volunteers, THE EXTRA MILE, FamilyCares, Seasons of Service, Kids Care Clubs, and MissionFish.

In 1988, Debbie Spaide got her children and their friends involved in community service, and the idea of kids serving spread in her community. She founded Kids Care in Connecticut and grew it into a large organization involving 75,000 kids and 1,400 registered Kids Care Clubs in the United States, Canada, Europe, Africa, and Asia. While Debbie and her able staff are still involved, Kids Care was taken over and is run by Points of Light Foundation, which is now under Michelle Nunn and HandsOn leadership.

A 1996 *Independent Sector* study shows that one in three teens started volunteering before age 14; teens were four times more likely to volunteer if they were asked; and 70% of teens who volunteered reported it was important because it gave them a new perspective, allowing them to do something important for a cause. A 1993 *Search Institute* study also found that young people who engage in two hours of service per week are half as likely to engage in high-risk behavior such as fights, truancy, smoking, drinking, and drug use.

Just two hours of service a week bolsters resiliency, improves self-esteem, increases personal responsibility and connects young people to others.

Light a candle, send a flicker of hope, shine bright in the darkness and call:

Points of Light Foundation & HandsOn Network

1875 K Street, NW, Fifth Floor

Washington, DC 20006

Phone: (202) 729-8000

E-mail: info@pointsoflight.org

OR 600 Means Street, Suite 210

Atlanta, Georgia 30318

Phone: (404) 979-2900 | Fax: (404) 979-2901

E-mail: info@handsonnetwork.org

Website: www.handsonnetwork.org

Kids Care Clubs, Points of Light & Hands On Network

975 Boston Post Road

Darien, Connecticut 06820

Phone: (203) 656-8052 | Toll Free: (866) 269-0510

Fax: (203) 656-8062

E-mail: kidscare@pointsoflight.org

Website: www.kidscare.org

CELEBRATING PASSIONARIES
IN BUSINESS

*"Whether you think you can
or you think you can't,
you're right."*
—Henry Ford

*"Achievement seems to be connected with action.
Successful men and women keep moving.
They make mistakes, but they don't quit."*
—Conrad Hilton

*"The best way to predict the future
is to create it."*
—Peter Drucker

*"Somehow I can't believe
that there are any heights
that can't be scaled by a man
who knows the secrets
of making dreams come true.
This special secret,
it seems to me, can be summarized in four C s.
They are curiosity, confidence, courage, and constancy."*
—Walt Disney

A Salute to Business Passionaries

While there are too many extraordinary heroes in business to report, the following is a sampling of entrepreneurs and businesses we salute.

Pat Blum

The Corporate Angel Network

From Airplane Wings
to Angel Wings

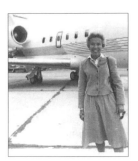

Life-changing ideas come in all shapes and sizes. Some arrive in tiny packages, like a hint or an intuition. The life-changing idea that hit Priscilla (Pat) Blum in 1981 was a little bigger. It was, literally, the size of a corporate jet.

In the cramped cockpit of her single-engine plane, waiting to take off, the 5'2", 100 pound Blum often found herself dwarfed by the corporate jets around her. As she looked out at the lines of sleek aircraft, which were used by companies to fly their employees to meetings, business engagements, and other trips, she noticed their corporate cabins were rarely full, often taking off with just a few passengers. Luggage, briefcases, or sports equipment occupied many of the seats—not people. She asked herself, "Why couldn't some of those empty seats be put to better use?"

Pat, who had fought and won a battle with breast cancer in 1969, was on the board of Connecticut's American Cancer Society. The society, which often helped cancer patients access specialized treatment, was frequently in a financial bind. Very few hospitals could provide bone marrow transplants, often crucial for saving the lives of leukemia patients. The best facility was in Seattle, clear across the country from where Pat lived. Many patients, already paying for costly medical care, just couldn't afford frequent flights to the West Coast. At cancer society meetings, she and other members would rack their brains, trying to come up with ways to help their cash-strapped patients get to the best hospitals.

One day, in the middle of a board meeting, Pat had a brainstorm. "Maybe some corporations could be persuaded to take cancer patients with them—using the empty seats on their plane—if the plane was going at the right time to a place the patient needed to go." Pat said her colleagues on the board thought she had lost her mind, but they told her it was worth researching. So Pat went to work.

From a makeshift "mission control center" in her home, her plan took off. Corporate planes would continue to operate on the same schedules without any interruptions or liabilities, and merely give a lift to the cancer patient, who might be accompanied by a companion if space was available. Then, with enthusiastic help from her friend and fellow cancer survivor, Jay Weinberg, they developed a strategy. Pat and Jay went directly to top corporate leaders who espoused social responsibility and invited them to "put their jets where their mouths were." With this, Corporate Angel Network (CAN) was launched.

To Pat and Jay's delight and to the initial surprise of their American Cancer Society colleagues, dozens of Fortune 500 corporations agreed to get on board. These public-spirited companies became an honor-roll of "angels" who were the first to join the network. They provide free, comfortable, and stress-free transportation for cancer patients traveling to hospitals all over the United States. After seeing Pat's brilliant idea becoming reality, Jay once said sheepishly, "I wonder why I didn't think of that?"

Twenty years later, CAN and its more than 500 companies fly an average of 150 patients each month to hospitals and treatment centers throughout the nation. This allows patients to avoid expensive, often inconvenient commercial flights and to travel in the dignity and comfort of corporate jets. And it's not just corporations with airplanes that have gotten in on the act. Dozens of limousine companies and hotels also have offered their complimentary services and rooms to the network.

"The passion was contagious," Pat said. "One thing just led to another."

Today, CAN and its corporate partners have found a way for thousands of cancer patients, bone marrow donors, and family members to fly, stay, and ride for free while undergoing cancer treatment or participating in important clinical drug trials. The program is open to all patients who do not require a doctor's care or any special en route services while traveling. Eligibility is based on medical need, not financial need, and patients and their families may use the service as often as necessary.

While Pat and Jay are both retired and no longer at the helm, CAN still runs smoothly. With about 60 volunteers and five paid staffers, this organization works with the flight departments of approximately 500 corporations to arrange about 1,200 flights per year, creating what Pat calls a "combination of public good and private enterprise." Without the network and its *gratis* travel accommodations, several clinical trials for cancer drugs might never have been possible, because sufficient numbers of patients could not have been enrolled.

Perhaps one of the most striking features of CAN and its participating companies is the lack of fanfare that accompanies their good deeds. The network operates day in day out, with a minimum of media attention. Not a single corporate "good samaritan" has ever sought public acclaim. This low profile is mandated in part by the desire for corporate security, but many companies forego public relations campaigns for another reason: They have flown so many flights that helping people in need has become second nature. For CAN's 500 corporations and their thousands of employees, being good citizens is a civic responsibility, not something to brag about.

As the "angel" network has grown, so have operating costs. The deliberate lack of public attention to CAN often forced Pat to find creative ways of raising money for computers and staffers. Through the generosity of one volunteer's relative, a Washington-based, aviation-oriented group holds an annual golf tournament to benefit CAN, raising more than $100,000 each year. Many other like-minded foundations and charities around the country also have been successfully tapped to donate the necessary funds.

Now in her late 70s, Pat has spent many years stumping for money at dinner parties. With her passion for the project and her personal experience with cancer, she has convinced hundreds of donors to be engaged, ensuring that CAN continues to turn airplane wings into angel wings.

"Anyone with an idea—whether it is tiny and local or as big as a national flight program—can change the world for the better," Pat said. "All it takes is the determination to validate the idea, a little planning, a lot of commitment, and the resolve to jump in with both feet and both hands."

From CAN . . . by Pat Blum

Pat remembers one particular young family in which both parents struggled with blindness. "They touched me deeply because they put up such a brave front and were so very courageous," Pat said. "Surely it was a dreadful burden for both parties in a marriage to be blind and then to have their very young child also blinded by eye cancer—it just seemed like an unbearable load." CAN was overjoyed to help.

The couple never complained and was extremely grateful to CAN. "If we couldn't find a flight to get them and their daughter to a specialist across the country, they never showed any frustration," Pat recalled. "The family had just one request: to make sure that their guide dog, Shadow, could travel with them. Initially, Pat thought corporations would hesitate, but was thrilled that none of the dozens of corporations who flew this very special family ever voiced an objection to bringing Shadow on board.

"It broke everyone's heart at CAN when these treasured friends phoned one day to say that, after several years and many flights for treatments, their daughter had lost her battle with cancer," Pat said. "A couple of years after this tragedy, the father contacted us to say that he and his wife were in the process of adopting another child. During the years that they traveled with us, we all became deeply attached to this family, as did every flight department and every executive who ever met them."

Thanks to the generosity of more than 500 of America's finest corporations, Corporate Angel Network has arranged thousands upon thousands of flights since Pat Blum founded CAN in 1981. It continues to help more than 150 patients a month.

Be a Corporate Angel... Your company can join more than 500 major corporations and use an empty seat on your aircraft traveling on routine business to give a cancer patient a lift to life-saving, state-of-the-art cancer treatment at no cost or inconvenience to you.

Patient Info... Call the Corporate Angel Network's toll-free Patient Line at (866) 328-1313 to register within three weeks of a specific appointment at a recognized cancer treatment center.

Want to give a cancer patient a lift? Want to help? Contact:

The Corporate Angel Network, Inc.

Westchester County Airport

One Loop Road

White Plains, New York 10604-1215

Phone: (914) 328-1313 | Fax: (914) 328-3938

E-mail: info@corpangelnetwork.org

Website: www.corpangelnetwork.org

Jim and Jeff Morgan are a remarkable father-son combination. Each has taken his separate path in life, and both benefit humanity in special ways. They represent business passionaries serving humanity. This first story profiles the father, Jim.

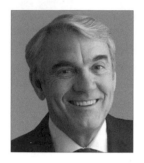

Jim Morgan
The Nature Conservancy

From Redwood Forests
to Grains of Sand

"I've always been interested in the outdoors and taking the kids camping, hiking, and river rafting. Winding down from Applied Materials and getting out of being CEO, I thought that I wanted to spend more time on the environmental community. I felt I needed to give back." —Jim Morgan

If you have a personal computer on your desk or in your briefcase, you should thank Jim Morgan. As chairman of Applied Materials, Jim has been hugely responsible for the way we live today—the company creates and sells the technology that makes the integrated circuit inside your computer. And the technology that makes your new flat-screen television "flat" likely started with Applied Materials as well. It's an internationally acclaimed, cutting-edge Silicon Valley success story.

Jim Morgan's vision is broader than building Applied Materials into the world's largest semiconductor equipment company and leading producer of nano (very tiny) manufacturing technology. It also includes concern for Giant Redwood trees and deserts through his involvement with The Nature Conservancy.

Growing up in an Indiana farm town of just a few hundred people, Jim gleaned values that became the foundation of his life. He loved nature and the feel of dirt under his bare feet, as well as the way the town took care of its own. "It was individuals helping individuals," Jim shares. "Even from the early days, I always felt I needed to give back. My personal mission in life and at Applied Materials became helping people and organizations meet their full potential."

Since Jim joined Applied Materials in its early years, revenues went from about $22 million a year in 1976 to just under $10 billion in 2007. Jim also has guided the company in recognizing the importance of social responsibility—and leading the way in places where they do business. "A couple of years after I got to Applied Materials, we decided we would fund 1% of our pre-tax profit into giving back and have been doing it ever since," Jim said. "I was always a venture capitalist and could see that planting seed money could make a big difference. We gave our time, energy, and resources where they could do the most good, acting on our belief that making a social contribution is defined not by who we are, but by what we do."

Through business and community efforts, Applied Materials and its employees seek to improve the quality of life in the world they share. That includes employees reaching out to underserved people in their area. It also means pioneering exciting "green" technologies. The company recently entered the solar photovoltaic equipment market, with a strategy to bring significant change to the industry by enabling lower cost-per-watt solutions for solar cell manufacturing, and a goal of making solar power a significant alternative source of global energy.

In 2000, Jim was one of the early supporters creating The Tech Awards: Technology Benefiting Humanity, an international program based at San Jose, California's Tech Museum. Each year they recognize innovators from around the world who are applying technology to serve humanity. To date, 175 entrepreneurial laureates have been honored, with winners receiving awards totaling $1,750,000.

In 2004, Jim was presented with the program's first Global Humanitarian Award, honoring individuals whose broad vision and leadership address humanity's greatest challenges. Subsequent winners of this award, which later became known as the James C. Morgan Global Humanitarian Award, include passionaries such as:

♥ Kristine Pearson, executive director of the FreePlay Foundation
♥ Microsoft co-founder and chairman Bill Gates
♥ Intel co-founder and technology luminary, Gordon Moore

♥ Professor Muhammad Yunus, whose Grameen Bank has allowed rural poor in Bangladesh to get microcredit loans to buy livestock and weaving materials

On the opposite spectrum of technology, Jim balances his love of the environment as an enthusiastic board member of The Nature Conservancy (TNC). This global nonprofit organization works around the world to preserve ecologically important lands and waters for nature and people. Reflecting on his childhood love of the land, Jim said: "I've always been interested in the outdoors and taking the kids camping and hiking or going river rafting. As I was transitioning at Applied Materials from CEO to chairman, I wanted to spend more time helping the environmental community." As a trustee of The Nature Conservancy of California, he saw a need to preserve and protect Redwood trees, deserts, and high mountains in the state. Later, he was elected to the Asia-Pacific Council, advising The Nature Conservancy's global board on its expansion in Asia. More recently, he became a member of the international board of directors.

"I believe business leaders and corporations can and should play a vital role in identifying and extending the benefits of technology to those who need them most."

It is easy to see the why Jim is attracted to The Nature Conservancy. Since its incorporation in 1951, the organization has protected more than 117 million acres of land and 5,000 miles of rivers worldwide, operating more than 100 marine conservation projects globally. With more than 1 million members, it works in all 50 states and in more than 30 countries, protecting habitats from grasslands to coral reefs.

Spanning the globe from Alaska to Zambia, the organization addresses threats to conservation involving climate change, fire, fresh water, forests, and invasive species, as well as marine ecosystems. Using a science-based approach to conservation, more than 700 staff scientists pursue non-confrontational, pragmatic solutions to the ecological challenges.

As a businessman, Jim knows the advantages of partnerships. The Nature Conservancy works with communities, businesses, governments, multilateral institutions, indigenous communities, as well as other nonprofit organizations to accomplish its goals. "One of the projects we're pulling together is a strategy for the Northern Sierras that covers all aspects of forest, water, development, conservation, and education," he explained. "We use science to select areas which have the most biodiversity and movement of habitat, including watershed areas. Over 60% of California water comes from the Northern Sierra, and that area is the most efficient carbon conversion area in the world. Plus, it's a wonderful place to have recreation."

In career and philanthropy, Jim likes to show that technology, science, and focus can unleash the potential in all of us and turn ideas into solutions for a better world. "The early founders of Silicon Valley, like the founders of Intel and Hewlett Packard, made a lot of money, but were not motivated by capital as much as their mission to take an idea and make something great happen," he said. "I believe business leaders and corporations can and should play a vital role in identifying and extending the benefits of technology to those who need them most."

Whether it is through Applied Materials, The Tech Awards, the Morgan Family Foundation, or The Nature Conservancy, Jim Morgan is a true venture capitalist who plants seed money to grow solutions for the challenges facing our world.

Becky Morgan and the Morgan Family Foundation

Jim Morgan brought along more than family values when he moved from the farmlands of Indiana to the high-tech world of Silicon Valley in 1968. He also brought his wife, Becky, who used her talents to represent California as a State Senator, then went on to become president of the Joint Venture Silicon Valley Network, a nonprofit organization of business, government, and education leaders. For years, Becky has served on the board of trustees for Cornell University where she and Jim attended, and has been a member of the President's Council of Cornell Women.

Fabulous credentials and accomplishments like these don't tell Becky Morgan's whole story, however. The mother of two also heads the Morgan Family Foundation, a first-rate example of the power of family foundations—a growing phenomenon that now numbers more than 37,000 and collectively granted more than $16 billion in 2006.

"Our desire to give back stems from our gratitude for our good fortune and our belief that those who are so blessed have a unique responsibility to help others," Becky said. "We believe that whether wealth is earned or inherited, it is important to help others and to do our part to leave some part of the world better than we found it."

The Morgan Family Foundation is a family endeavor that seeks to make a difference by helping individuals and organizations reach their full potential. Jim and Becky's two adult children and their spouses sit on the board, and together shape the foundation's mission and values.

"Our shared goal is to see a return on our investment measured by lives changed and communities transformed," Becky shares. "The impact of our philanthropy will be seen in young people reaching their educational goals and making responsible life choices, in protecting open spaces and cultural heritage sites, and in managing issues by regional stewards through collaboration.

It is important to us that the second and third generations (our children and grandchildren) demonstrate generosity and experience the hard work, the time commitment, and the joy of giving to those who use our gifts wisely," she continues. "We end our Values Statement with 'Generosity is contagious and should be encouraged in others.' We are proud of the work of the Morgan Family Foundation and encourage all families with resources beyond life's necessities to give back, whatever their areas of interest."

For More Information

The Nature Conservancy, incorporated in 1951, is the world's leading environmental organization, helping to protect the most ecologically important lands and waters around the world for nature and for people. Highly rated by *The Charity Navigator* for efficiency, capacity, and financial health, this international nonprofit organization has protected more than 117 million acres of land and 5,000 miles of rivers worldwide. It operates more than 100 marine conservation projects globally. With more than 1 million members, The Nature Conservancy works in all 50 states and in more than 30 countries, protecting habitats from grasslands to coral reefs.

Adopt an Acre; Rescue a Reef; Go Green; and support Mother Nature effectively. Contact:

The Nature Conservancy, Worldwide Office

4245 North Fairfax Drive, Suite 100

Arlington, Virginia 22203-1606

Phone: (800) 628-6860

Website: www.nature.org

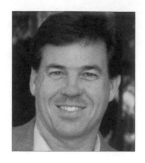

Jeff Morgan
Global Heritage Fund

Saving World Heritage
One Site at a Time

"We had a vision from the beginning that we were not going to be a one-trick pony."
                                                                    –Jeff Morgan

If you enjoyed the "National Treasure" movies, then you might think of Jeff Morgan as a Nicholas Cage for the world.

As executive director of the nonprofit Global Heritage Fund (GHF), Jeff leads a mission to preserve and protect humanity's most important archaeological and cultural treasures in developing countries. His vision takes him on quests like saving ancient ruins in Iraq, creating the largest national park in Guatemala, and protecting historic villages in China threatened by looting, lumbering, neglect, and urban sprawl. With 14 projects underway or in development, Jeff works with local governments to re-discover and value jewels like the Hampi ruins in India, the My Son temple in Vietnam, the Wat Phou temple in Laos, and projects in Pakistan, Turkey, Libya, and Peru. Although GHF is only 5 years old, the organization is already a "multi-trick pony."

As the son of legendary technology leader Jim Morgan, Jeff worked in Silicon Valley as a software marketing specialist. "When I cashed out of my second high-tech start-up, I decided to switch careers and find something that would use my unique set of skills, which are working in language and culture," Jeff stated. "There are 40 large wildlife-nature preservation groups worldwide, and yet nobody was focused on restoring endangered heritage sites, especially in the developing world. Since there was a big hole with no one filling it, I 'volunteered.' "

In 2002, the 45-year-old Stanford MBA and father of three switched gears to create the Global Heritage Fund. "From high tech to low tech, it is all the same skills," Jeff said. "In marketing, I was always working overseas and had learned four foreign languages (Mandarin, Japanese, French, and Spanish), as well as how to deal with people of different cultures." He also was well connected in the world of international finance and trade. Perfectly positioned, Jeff began his odyssey.

His first stop was traveling to Petra, Jordan, the ancient, rock-carved city whose temple was featured in the movie "Indiana Jones and the Last Crusade." When he found that tourism to Petra was the No. 1 industry in the whole country, he realized the potential economic benefit of preservation. Traveling to ancient cultural landmarks that were crumbling into ruin, Jeff logged about 144,000 air miles each of his first few years. He saw how restoring these sites could jump-start economic engines in country after country.

Jeff's initial foray into southwest China was the 1,000-year-old city of Lijiang. "This area was being destroyed by unplanned modern development, and China had two people sipping tea as their management group," Jeff recalled. "We put them through our unique step-by-step process called 'Preservation By Design' and created a master plan, then worked with them in a scientific conservation process. We helped the leaders create a financial funding base model so they could achieve long term sustainability for their projects."

For Lijiang, GHF raised funds in Palo Alto, California, and the local Chinese government matched the money. "It was exciting to see some local Chinese in California thrilled to invest back in their own country, comfortable knowing they had an audited U.S. nonprofit managing the restoration, without corruption," Jeff said. The fact they were working with a professional international partner–GHF–enabled the local Chinese government to get funds from national offices in Beijing.

Although many historical sites in China were being decimated for new construction, GHF was instrumental in transforming Lijiang–one of China's last ancient towns–into a major tourist attraction. In just three years, the annual number of tourists grew from 300,000 to 800,000. In the process, many of the native Naxi families were profoundly affected as sanitation, sewage systems, water quality, construction, and preservation were improved. Success in Lijiang led to other Chinese projects, including the 1,200-year-old Foguang Temple, China's last building made entirely of wood, right down to the nails.

In GHF's second year, Jeff expanded to six projects, using the venture capital model of scaling up to raise capital. El Mirador in Guatemala–a new 600,000-acre national park–was the largest project. "This is very important for us, combining Mayan ruins with Maya biosphere, along with saving jaguar and wildlife habitat," Jeff shares. Opposing loggers and slash-and-burn farmers, GHF fought to save the area's 26 ruins, expand park boundaries, and develop this region as a tourist attraction. Mel Gibson's movie "Apocalypto" helped bring visitor attention to this area, which is known for unbroken jungle guarded by howler monkeys and snakes, as well as its magnificent 2,000-year-old pyramid. Tourism at El Mirador has grown from 300 to 3,200 annually, and GHF has helped El Mirador apply for recognition as a United Nations Educational, Scientific and Cultural Organization (UNESCO) World Heritage Site.

Since launching GHF in 2002, Jeff has put together a worldwide network of more than 600 archeologists, preservation experts, anthropologists, antiquities conservators, structural engineers, and other specialists to guide long-term planning, training, and restoration efforts. His strategy is to develop partnerships with donors, local governments, entrepreneurs, and conservation interests to work exclusively in developing countries, where GHF grants can go far. With the necessary infrastructure and accessibility, local economies can flourish, benefiting people in surrounding areas, some of whose annual incomes are less than $1,000 per person.

"We put them through our unique step-by-step process called 'Preservation By Design' and created a master plan, then worked with them in a scientific conservation process."

The high-energy, fast-talking, fully focused Jeff Morgan operates GHF with a full-time staff of only six employees from a small Victorian office building in downtown Palo Alto. With 14 sites worldwide, he travels to remote locations often reachable only on foot or by horseback. He has raised awareness and funding, leveraging more than $10 million to save and protect ruins. He creates opportunities for residents living near precious treasures like the lost monuments of the Champra Kingdom which ruled My Son, Vietnam, from the fourth to 13th centuries, and the ancient city of Kars in eastern Turkey, which dates back to the Ottoman Empire.

Iraq might be ravaged by war, but it also is home to ancient biblical cities such as Babylon, Nineveh, and Ur. With support from GHF to restore glorious antiquities, Jeff foresees the possibility of a stable Iraq using tourism as a new economic front to bolster its oil-based economy.

GHF is working with Iraqi leaders to save Aqar Quf, a 3,400-year-old city believed to be the capital of the ancient Kassite Dynasty.

Working with foreign governments is part of Jeff's calling. While some Chinese businessmen are willing to destroy ancient sites for the sake of money, Chinese cultural leaders are highly educated and deeply passionate about the historical relevance of their dynasties. "If they have the funding and get a bit of help from us, they can do better conservation than almost anybody." Jeff added, "And the Japanese are very culturally adept. In Peru, they gave us $4 million to build a museum and have helped us build a new visitor's center in Laos."

Jeff doesn't see old ruins as just interesting tourist spots. "They tend to be economic engines for their regions," he said. "They provide growth, jobs, and long-term income for the people who live there." In the end, though, Global Heritage Fund sites depend on the skills and determination of local people, as well as the generosity of those committed to helping conserve our world's ancient legacies.

For Jeff, who majored in urban planning as an undergraduate in the College of Architecture, Art, and Planning at Cornell University, life has come full circle. He has traveled through the world of cutting-edge technology and come back to city planning—saving the history of our global treasures.

For More Information

Founded in 2002 by Jeff Morgan, Global Heritage Fund is an international conservancy dedicated to protecting archaeological sites and ancient townscapes in developing countries. In preserving humanity's most important treasures, Global Heritage Fund invests capital, assembles a global network of experts, and works with governments protecting cultural heritage sites. They have developed a unique and holistic "Preservation By Design" methodology to achieve sustainable conservation, training, economic development, and funding for 14 sites worldwide, including Peru, Guatemala, Turkey, Iraq, Libya, Laos, Cambodia, China, India, Pakistan and Vietnam. For those who wish to invest in protecting the treasures of the past for our future, GHF offers targeted trips and the adventure of a lifetime.

Grab your fedora, climb aboard, and help protect our world's heritage treasures! Contact:

Global Heritage Fund

625 Emerson Street, Suite 200

Palo Alto, California 94301

Phone: (650) 325-7520 | Fax (650) 325-7511

E-mail: info@globalheritagefund.org

Website: www.globalheritagefund.org

> *"Many small people*
> *who in many small places*
> *doing many small things*
> *can change the face of the world"*
> *—graffiti on the Berlin Wall*

Paul Brainerd and Friends...
Social Venture Partners

Fostering Positive Local Impact

After selling his Aldus Corporation to Adobe Systems, Inc., entrepreneur Paul Brainerd launched into a career as a philanthropist. For almost a year, he traveled throughout the United States with his assistant Bonni Alpert researching various models of giving. His goal was to put together a model of philanthropy that combined traditional philanthropic approaches with more innovative methods of giving that would appeal to a new generation of people.

Paul was excited to see a growing interest among nonprofits to establish deeper relationships with financial supporters, to increase access to business skills, and to focus a greater amount of energy on building organizational infrastructure. "Once I had some ideas together," recalled Brainerd, "I then enlisted some co-conspirators—people in the community who had already demonstrated an interest in giving back in various areas." Included in this group were business leaders Doug Walker, CEO of the software firm Walker, Richer and Quinn (WRQ), Bill Neukom, former Executive Vice President and General Counsel for Microsoft, and two former Microsoft vice presidents, Ida Cole and Scott Oki. "We combined our Rolodexes, and we planned an event," said Brainerd. "One-hundred-thirty-six people came to our Seattle gathering that evening, and in 1997 Social Venture Partners (SVP) was formed."

Brainerd shared his original concept for SVP Seattle, "What we looked for are great people with good ideas who can make an impact on the social problems in our community...there are many people out there with incredible ideas. Few have had all the training and support they need in order to be really successful."

Using the venture capital approach as a model, they created the concept of donors—**partners**—who would not only contribute financially, but would offer their time and expertise to build long-term partnerships with nonprofit organizations—**investees**. By the end of summer 1997, nearly 40 individuals or couples had signed on as partners, agreeing to donate $5,000 each year and actively participate in the activities of the organization for at least two years (couples that join together are considered a single entity). Throughout the partnership, measuring outcomes would be a high priority. "Perhaps the goal of measuring outcomes stems from a bias we have, given our background in the business world," said Brainerd. "Nonetheless, we think that focusing on outcomes not only benefits us as investors, it also benefits the nonprofits."

According to founder Paul Brainerd, the core of the SVP model appealed to a new younger generation of people. "...the traditional approach of writing a check to a charitable organization or serving on a board did not seem fulfilling enough. There was a desire to be more engaged in the process of giving back." SVP Partners not only write a check but also are encouraged to contribute their time, expertise and provide whatever resources it takes for the success of their nonprofit beneficiaries. They contribute in areas such as mentoring, information technology, financial management, strategic planning, fund development, legal, marketing, and more.

Ten years have since passed and the dual mission of SVP remains unchanged. The organization seeks to be both an engaged grant-maker as well as a catalyst for individual giving. Their mission is simple: advance the common good by engaging and connecting a community of philanthropic business leaders to strengthen local nonprofits. They reasoned that as a community of Partners, they could leverage their combined financial and human capital to create more value than they could as individuals and could collaborate with nonprofits and philanthropic organizations that had compatible goals.

Today, more than 420 local Seattle Partners contribute their know-how, resources, and passion to more than 20 King County nonprofit organizations. Learning from each other and the groups they support, Partners have provided over 75,000 hours of volunteer consulting and have granted in excess of $10 million to advance promising nonprofits in their area.

The local accomplishments of SVP have inspired others to do the same. As of April 2007, there are 23 SVP organizations and over 1,000 total Partnerships across North America, with investments ranging from $2,770 to $35,000, and new Affiliates springing up across the globe.

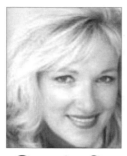

San Diego Social Venture Partners

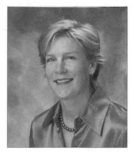

Carrie Stone   ## Darcy Bingham

Darcy Bingham and Carrie Stone were strangers whose lives paralleled until their paths accidently crossed, enabling them to co-found the San Diego Social Venture Partners (SDSVP). In 2001 Carrie Stone, a single mother and successful San Diego businesswoman in her mid forties, had never heard of SVP, but she had trodden the well-worn working path and acquired plenty of stuff that provided little meaning. "I wanted to be less self absorbed so I took a life-break to explore a healthy balance between self and others. I wanted to give back but wanted to do it in an intimate personal way," said Carrie. Her eight-year-old son Ben was already mastering the art of philanthropy under his mother's guidance, giving away one third of his pocket money. "Ben joined Kids Korps which engaged him in hands-on local philanthropy and helping others with projects like pet therapy with seniors and building homes in Mexico. I could see these experiences became real to him and also to me. That was exactly what I was looking for so I began looking into venture philanthropy."

Darcy and Bob Bingham had just sold a successful company during the high-tech boom in 1998. The young couple, then in their early thirties, were reassessing their life path and looking for the right causes. "We were very young and fortunate because causes had yet to pick us," said Darcy. "We were on an exploration mission when the San Diego Foundation (SDF) asked me to join their board." The SDF is a leading San Diego resource for information about charitable giving and community needs working with philanthropists to develop creative solutions to meet those critical needs.

In her new board role, Darcy attended a Foundations Conference and heard a presentation by Seattle's SVP Executive Director Paul Shoemaker. "There was a panel discussing this new venture capital model where partners actively nurture their financial investments with guidance and resources. Investing time, expertise and money into nonprofits was a very entrepreneurial idea and Seattle was promoting a kind of SVP in a box, a how-to start a SVP in your city. It lit a fire under me and I thought—why don't we have one in San Diego?"

"Our Partners hungered to make an impact by being more hands-on, leveraging their talents and gifts within the organizations we invested in."

Fate took a hand when Darcy Bingham and Carrie Stone bumped into each other upon leaving a local event. Together they walked to the parking lot where they spent an hour discussing their dreams and passions around philanthropy. The encounter culminated in them joining forces and founding San Diego Social Venture Partners. "Everything about SVP fit our personal values and desires to find a better way to invest our charitable dollars. We also got lucky because The San Diego Foundation was willing to help us by sharing their expertise," explained Darcy. "We held a party and recruited our friends, educators and entrepreneurs who shared an important trait: to know what you don't know and find people who do." Darcy and Carrie also noticed that SDSVP attracted people of similar value systems, people with a pay-it-forward ideal.

"It was not always easy in the early days," said Carrie. "This new model of giving that was focused on ROI—a return on the investment that was measurable from an impact perspective—was somewhat novel and also threatening to some. We passionately believed that philanthropy and donating to charities needed to move well beyond writing a check.

"We call our investors partners. Our partners hungered to make an impact by being more hands-on, leveraging their talents and gifts within the organizations we invested in. Their giving became more experiential and meaningful. Each year they choose a different focus area for grants. In 2006–2007, SDSVP supported organizations delivering services focused on hunger and homelessness in San Diego. Previous investment cycles have concentrated on Early Childhood Development, the Environment, Employment and Economic Development, Health and

Human Services and Education, all with a goal to create opportunities for self-sufficiency."

According to Darcy and Carrie, many partners have spread their philanthropy arteries beyond SVP by establishing funds at The San Diego Foundation or becoming board members of their nonprofit beneficiaries. "This is one wonderful ripple effect of the organization and we have watched it extend to our investees and beneficiaries," said Stone.

SDSVP has grown to over 140 partners, and over the last five years has worked with 10 different Investees, contributing an estimated $5.6 million in cash and in-kind services which includes more than 17,000 strategic and volunteer hours. The other blessing is the personal relationships and friendships that have developed among partners with like values that may have never met each other otherwise. Carrie has expanded her focus globally, working to show her teen son Ben that the world needs more young humanitarians. They will travel to Kenya with "Free the Children" to build schools and learn more about Kenya development initiatives from a holistic perspective. Carrie shares, "I feel immensely blessed to have played a small role in being a catalyst for philanthropic change in the San Diego region."

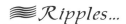 *Ripples...*

Eva Pacheco

One example of San Diego SVP is a three-year grant made in April 2002 to Excellence and Justice in Education (EJE). The grant allowed this parent involvement group to expand services and open a center to educate Hispanic parents about their rights and responsibilities to advocate for educating their children, both in the classroom and with the school administration. "Being ill-informed parents directly affects their children's ability to succeed in school and later in life," said EJE founder Eva Pacheco.

Two years ago, the untimely closing of a local district school servicing mostly low-income children of Mexican origin provided EJE the chance to birth their total vision and mission. With a proactive ideology that stems from love of children, they opened EJE Elementary Academy, a charter school using the Dual Language (English/Spanish) Immersion

Model highlighting the value of diversity, curriculum accessibility and a provision of equal educational opportunities. "Many times second language and low-income students get lost in the system and are not provided with the tools to grow, learn and develop," said Eva. "At 15 and 16 years of age they often leave school with poor reading and writing skills and a lack of motivation."

Not surprisingly, Eva Pacheco is Executive Director of the charter school and works together with a SDSVP partner, co-chairing the Board of Trustees. The school is K–5 with 12 classrooms and 240 children, and they are currently revising their charter with the school district to expand to grades K–8, comprised of a K–5 Elementary Academy, and grades 6–8 Middle School Academy, each with an estimated 400 children.

"The success of our school is driven by its teachers, board members, parents, administrators, community volunteers and EJE supporters like SDSVP. All are committed to developing children who will be good role models in the community—good citizens. Our academic program is only part of the solution," said Pacheco. "We strive for long-term success so that achievement is not only academic but develops into a way of life that continues for a lifetime."

"Working together,
ordinary people can perform
extraordinary feats.
They can push things that come into their hands
a little higher up,
a little farther on
towards the heights of excellence."
—B. J. Marshall

For More Information

In 1997, entrepreneur Paul Brainerd and friends including Scott Oki and Ida Cole created Social Venture Partners (SVP) in Seattle with the goal of creating a better, more efficient, more business-like model to generate success in nonprofits. With an involved commitment of 2–3 years, their business-oriented partners invest both money and their expertise with a variety of growing nonprofits to ensure success. Established in 2001 by Darcy Bingham and Carrie Stone, the San Diego Social Venture Partners has pioneered a new form of giving in San Diego—venture philanthropy. Over the last 5 years SDSVP has worked with 10 different Investees, contributed an estimated $5.6 million in cash and in kind services which includes more than 17,000 strategic and volunteer hours. The SVP program has spread to 23 cities in the United States and is now international, enhancing the goals and visions of worthy nonprofits around the world.

San Diego Social Venture Partners

c/o The San Diego Foundation

2508 Historic Decatur Road, Suite 200

San Diego, California 92106

Phone for Becoming a Partner: (619) 235-2300

E-mail: sdsvp@sdfoundation.org

Social Venture Partners International

1601 Second Avenue, Suite 615

Seattle, Washington 98101

Phone: (206) 728-7872; Fax: (206) 728-0552

E-mail: info@svpi.org

Website: www.svpinternational.org

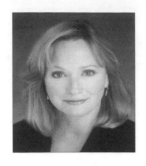

Susan Corrigan
Gifts in Kind International

A Closed Door Was Opportunity
Knocking

Susan Corrigan is the proud mother of three: a daughter, a son, and the eighth-largest charity in the United States. You may never have heard of Gifts In Kind International, but as a nonprofit it ranks just behind the American Red Cross. This nonprofit organization is the most extensive distributor of donated products in the world, and Susan Corrigan is the dynamic lady who created Gifts In Kind and steered its destiny for 23 years.

As assistant to the president of United Way of America in 1983, Susan found herself in an unusual situation. The 3M Corporation made a donation of $12 million in office supplies. Although more accustomed to receiving and distributing cash, the United Way leadership gratefully accepted the gift and then turned to Susan to manage the process of distributing it. Undaunted by the monumental task, Susan soon had the entire donation on its way to 600 enthusiastic local communities that had expressed a need for such items.

While the United Way leadership was interested in the concept of accepting donated products, they decided it did not fit in with their overall direction. Susan realized an exciting opportunity had landed in her lap, and she took a chance on a vision that seemed impossible.

In 1984, Susan left United Way and, with a grant from the Lilly Endowment, gave birth to Gifts In Kind. She also received support from William Ellinghaus, then president of AT&T. Susan and William recruited board members from some of the largest companies in the world, including Digital Equipment Corporation, Hewlett-Packard Development Company, IBM Corporation, JC Penney, Prudential Financial, RCA, 3M Corporation, Westinghouse Electric Corporation, and Xerox Corporation.

Since then, Susan's charity has generated more than $6.8 billion in manufactured product donations distributed through a network of more than 200,000 community charities and schools around the world. Providing assistance to millions of people, Gifts In Kind International's average annual growth rate has been a heady 35% a year, making it the fastest growing nonprofit with the lowest overhead in the United States. Amazingly, 99.7% of all donations go directly to communities and people in need. It is ranked as one of the most cost-efficient charities in the world.

Susan Corrigan has always worked hard and doesn't know any other way. At an early stage of her working life, she was putting together a television commercial and found herself working until 3 a.m. to beat a looming deadline. She decided that if she was going to put that much energy into her work, she wanted to make sure the product was something that would really make a difference in other people's lives. She decided to make the bold step of changing careers.

"It's difficult to always know if you're on the path that you're going to be on for the rest of your life," Susan said. "Sometimes it's hard to find that path. I worked at many jobs before Gifts In Kind, and I had great careers. I learned something at every job I've ever had and always strove for excellence. Young people should not assume that their first job is going to be exactly what they will do for life. There's a great deal of work involved in being successful at what you do."

Susan's deep need to help other people endure tough times was what led her to work for United Way in Chicago. She has spent the past 26 years feeling very fortunate to have been able to dedicate her life to serving others.

Susan's baby's nickname is "Product Philanthropy." And, like raising any child, it took many people to shape, plan, feed, encourage, and mentor her brainchild from its infancy. Gifts In Kind supporters now include many Fortune 500 corporations, as well as thousands of other smaller companies. In 2007, these companies generously donated nearly $900 million in new products.

"We don't want the organization to become an expensive roadblock between the donor company and the recipient charity," Susan explained, "so we operate on a budget of no more than 1% of the total value of what we distribute. Many good nonprofits have an operating budget of 15% to 25%. We are not only supporting a staff of 28 people with our 1%, but also shipping donations all over the world. Fortunately, we have great partners—corporations that work with us, such as transportation companies that provide free shipping. I believe success is a matter of involving as many people and organizations as possible in the grand idea of what it is you are trying to achieve."

Today's top manufacturers and retailers rely on Gifts In Kind International as a conduit for the donation of products, goods, and services from private corporations to the charitable sector, partnering with hundreds of major nonprofit agencies. On average, a charity receives $143 in new products for each $1 it provides to Gifts In Kind in registration and product distribution fees.

"Companies feel really good about contributing," Susan said, noting that "hiccups" in the marketing and distribution process often leave many manufacturers with large volumes of perfectly good inventory appropriate for donation. Companies look for worthy causes where their products can be put to good use in exchange for community goodwill, logistics cost savings, and tax breaks. Rather than having to find the charities, discuss the details, and deliver the goods themselves, companies turn to Gifts In Kind to handle it all, free of charge, any time of the year. As Susan shares, "It's always a good time to give."

"Corporate executives care just as much as anyone does about what's going on in their community, and they're looking for ways where they can be engaged and really make an impact."

Susan sees corporate executives as next-door neighbors, not as inhabitants of gray buildings on far-off hills. "They care just as much as anyone does about what's going on in their community, and they're looking for ways where they can be engaged and really make an impact," she said. "Gifts In Kind would not exist if it weren't for the overwhelming generosity of companies."

Susan has a big dream: that all corporations making or selling a product will include in their community involvement strategy a means for giving away products on an ongoing basis. "And if those products are given to the nonprofit sector so that vital community services are able to function at their highest level, it's a way to better the world," she said.

But having a vision is not all there is to success. Susan notes, "You not only have to have a dream, you have to have a plan as well. We have a 10-year strategic plan that we monitor on a daily basis. Everybody at Gifts In Kind understands their part in achieving those goals."

Meanwhile, Susan Corrigan is still looking to the future: "Many people look back on their lives and say they've accomplished certain things. But I look ahead and say I haven't done this yet, and I haven't done that, and there is so much more that needs to be done." Susan transitioned out of Gifts In Kind after 23 years as president, and now works with nonprofits and caring for her grandchildren. The organization, under the capable leadership of Barry Anderson, continues to flourish and do great work.

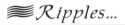 *Ripples...*

Red Nation Celebration

Gifts In Kind International in partnership with Toys 'R' Us and the Red Nation Celebration 2002, helped give away more than 400 toys to children on the Rose Bud Native American Reservation in South Dakota.

The toys were distributed in August as part of the 2002 Red Nation Celebration, an annual concert series that presents contemporary and traditional Native American music and dance to both Indian and non-Indian audiences.

"Through this donation," Susan said, "Gifts In Kind International is not only helping provide toys to underprivileged kids on the Rose Bud Reservation, but is also helping support promising Native American artists through our partnership with the Red Nation Celebration which was founded by Joanelle Romero." Joanelle said, "The children are our future and need to be cared for and honored. This is one way in which we can be of service to the future generations."

Sage Galesi, a 16-year-old Native American performer and the voice of youth on the Red Nation board of directors adds: "As a young person and a member of the board, I want to reinforce how important it is for corporate America to support the future generation. Organizations like Gifts In Kind International and Toys 'R' Us really make that happen, and I am proud to be part of this process."

Gifts In Kind International, founded in 1984 by Susan Corrigan, is the eighth largest nonprofit organization in the United States and the world's leading organization in "product philanthropy." Through 2004, under Ms. Corrigan's leadership, Gifts In Kind distributed $5.5 billion worth of quality new products and services—$900 million helping more than 13 million people in need in 2007 to 26 countries with a paid staff of just 28. Ranked as one of the most cost-efficient charities in the world, Gifts In Kind International operates at less than 1% of the total value of products, goods, and services contributed annually. Today's top manufacturers and retailers, including many Fortune 500 companies, rely on Gifts In Kind International to design and manage the donation process. In May 2005, Ms. Corrigan retired from the board after serving as founder and CEO for 23 years.

Gifts In Kind International is a network of more than 445 local affiliated partnerships in 26 countries around the world serving 150,000 deserving community charities. Contributions are made each year by 44% of Fortune 500 companies and thousands of corporations. Gifts In Kind International is looking for volunteers, which is a major factor in continuing an amazing .3% cost of operation, translating to 99.7% of all donations going directly to charity.

To be a kind superhero or super-corporate hero bearing incredible gifts, contact:

Gifts In Kind International

333 North Fairfax Street

Alexandria, Virginia 22314

Phone: (703) 836-2121 | Fax: (703) 798-3192

E-mail: registration@giftsinkind.org

Website: www.giftsinkind.org

Betty Mohlenbrock
United Through Reading

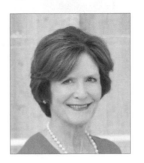

Uniting Deployed Service
Members & Their Children

In 1989, San Diego reading specialist, teacher, and mother, Betty Mohlenbrock was deeply concerned that so many children in this country couldn't read—and that one of the biggest reasons was the fact that parents weren't reading aloud with their kids. Studies showed that this simple activity was the single best way to secure a child's future academic success.

Having raised her own family, Betty also knew that reading together dramatically strengthened the bond between parent and child by providing a bridge for communication and sharing. Challenged to take action, Betty created United Through Reading (formerly called Family Literacy Foundation) with a lofty goal: to ensure that children from all backgrounds are read to regularly.

In 1991, Betty branched out even further with the United Through Reading Military Program, which videotaped deployed service members reading a children's book and then sent that DVD and the book back to their family. The initial trials proved that children at home loved cuddling up and hearing the sound of their mom or dad reading them a story over and over again as they watched the videos and read along. From there, it grew into a full-fledged quality-of-life program for military families, keeping parents and children connected while separated during long deployments.

> *Betty created United Through Reading (formerly called Family Literacy Foundation) with a lofty goal: to ensure that children from all backgrounds are read to regularly.*

The positive impact of the trials was so overwhelming that United Through Reading was soon adopted by the whole U.S. Navy. United Through Reading trained deployed personnel to manage the program while their ships were underway. These volunteers promoted the program, scheduled taping sessions, and provided coaching tips to participants. Homefront Coordinators also helped by creating shipboard libraries of children's books. Families who received the videotapes were encouraged to respond to the deployed loved one, sending letters, e-mail, or photographs of the child watching the video. They called this the "Full Circle Method of Communication."

The Navy raved about the program, and it soon spread to the Marines and beyond to other branches of the Armed Forces. The military recognized a huge dilemma: the most commonly cited grounds for leaving military service were the frequency of deployments and the subsequent effect on separated families.

General Peter Pace, former Chairman of the Joint Chiefs of Staff, wrote to Betty: "With characteristic heroism and spirit, our military families support these efforts while enduring extended deployments and separations. United Through Reading is an absolutely fantastic way to help service members and their loved ones stay connected in the face of such challenges."

Thousands of children and parents are feeling much closer to each other, and kids are less fearful about Mom or Dad's absence. Reunions are easier, morale is higher for everyone, and spouses at home enjoy the support of their deployed mates. One of the Homefront Coordinators (spouses at home promoting the program to other families) for the USS Anchorage shared, "It was incredible to watch my children's eyes light up. They started smiling and before I knew it, my son was talking back to the video as if his daddy was in the room with him. It was great!"

By 2007, Betty's United Through Reading program was benefiting more than 290,000 children and their parents by sending home "read aloud" DVDs. One story that especially touched Betty's heart was shared by a Homefront Coordinator for the USS Mobile Bay: "I personally have taken pictures and videotaped our children's responses to the DVD they received from their Sailor dad. Because it has been played over and over again, our son has much of the book memorized and recites it as he holds on to the books. Friends who have come over and witnessed this 'reading' of the book are amazed, not because he's only four-years-old, but because he's autistic and they can see he's enjoying each and every time he sees his dad on video."

"I will be sending a tape to their dad so he can see the effect he has on them, even while he's so far away. Recently, our son was watching the tape and moved a chair up to the TV so he could reach it, since it was high on the dresser. He first touched the screen, touching his dad's cheeks, and then he hugged the TV. He didn't say a word, but he didn't have to; his actions were enough. I e-mailed my husband and told him 'Keep them coming! He hears you, and he sees you, and he knows you love him!'" For a child with autism, it's harder to break through with a connection of love; for this family, it was a miracle.

Betty's strategy for reaching all deployed military personnel took a great stride forward when the White House notified her that Laura Bush had agreed to be Honorary Chair of the United Through Reading Military Program. She has now agreed to continue on for 2008–2009. Target Corporation has been a proud supporter of the military program for three years and is responsible for its expansion to all the Armed Forces. Diligence, determination, and a great idea have paid great dividends!

Can you see it through a child's eyes? Hearing and seeing the parent you miss so much, reading a book to you every day? Betty won't be satisfied until all deployed military personnel and their families realize this dream. A little bit of home brings a lot of hope and love to servicemen and women who are separated continents away from their families.

Betty and her dream of improving literacy and family communication have taken flight, soaring with precision accuracy toward accomplishing its "golden books" mission. United Through Reading has expanded their mission to also include a similar outreach to prison inmates and grandparents who want to remain close to the children they love.

In 1989, Betty Mohlenbrock created Family Literacy Foundation in San Diego to help end illiteracy, focusing on reading aloud to children. Family Literacy branched out in 1991 into what is now known as United Through Reading, which enables our overseas servicemen and women to be recorded reading a children's book that is sent to their children who miss them back at home. More than 412,000 parents, spouses and children have benefited from the nationally acclaimed United Through Reading's Military, Inmate and Grandparent programs.

Shape up or ship out! Support our military families through the power of reading. Contact:

United Through Reading

11555 Sorrento Valley Road, Suite 203

San Diego, California 92121

Phone: (858) 481-7323

Website: www.unitedthroughreading.org

"Believe it!
High expectations
are the key to everything."
—Sam Walton

Stan Smith
Boys & Girls Clubs of America

**Still Serving Aces,
Tennis Great Supports Kids**

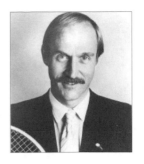

During the 1970s, Stan Smith was "Mr. Tennis." Named "Best Player in the World" in 1971, he followed that up by winning Wimbledon in 1972. During his playing career, he racked up 39 world singles tournament wins and another 61 world doubles titles, usually with his long-time partner, Bob Lutz. Smith played on the U.S. Davis Cup Team 11 times, bringing seven trophies home to the United States. He came back in the 1980s to win just about every trophy available for tennis players aged 35 and over. He has won a permanent, prominent place in the International Tennis Hall of Fame. Stan is just as well known for his sportsmanship and courteous behavior on and off the court.

Smith continued to serve his sport prestigiously in later years, first as the coaching director for the United States Tennis Association from 1988 to 1993, then as the Coach for the U.S. Men's Tennis Team at the Olympic Games in Sydney. Today, his company, Stan Smith Design, has created dozens of the top tennis facilities around the world. He also runs an "events company," Stan Smith Events, which helps corporations host clients at major sporting events. Stan is now probably best known nationally for his line of terrific tennis shoes, carried by Adidas. In 1971, he became the touring tennis pro of Sea Pines Resort in Hilton Head Island, South Carolina, where he, his wife, Margie and their four children make their home

Throughout his life, Stan Smith felt his athletic achievements were not enough to fulfill his purpose in life. Yearning to meaningfully exercise his Christian calling, he has always had a special place in his heart for reaching out to disadvantaged youth. "I was with my dad at a Kiwanis International Club meeting and this guy spoke from Big Brothers. I went up to him afterwards and asked if it was possible to start a chapter at college. He said it hadn't been done, but there's no reason why we couldn't. So with the support of my fraternity brothers in Beta Theta Pi, I started a chapter for Big Brothers of America at the University of Southern California (USC) where I went to college," Stan said. "We had a dozen guys in the Beta house that would spend a couple of hours a week with 'little brothers' assigned to them from the neighboring area of Watts."

Stan fondly recalls his own "little brother," Cliff, who was full of life. "He was also from the Watts area. We would go out and play catch or go bowling—just doing activities for an hour. Then I'd take Cliff home. He didn't have a father and his mother worked. We developed a relationship that meant a lot to both of us."

Although his tennis career intervened over the next couple of decades, Stan never lost his vision for being involved with youngsters. "When the people directing the Boys & Girls Club in Hilton Head approached me years later, I realized the way the organization worked was the best vehicle for youngsters to get out of the rut they're in," he said. "Boys & Girls Clubs reach out to a lot of kids who don't have two parents or come from disadvantaged or dysfunctional families, or possibly are headed in the wrong direction."

Stan went from supporter to spokesperson and fundraiser for the Boys & Girls Club in his hometown. "We now have a beautiful facility including a gym with basketball and volleyball courts, a recreation room with pool tables, a craft area, music room and a library. We also have a wing just for computer instruction where the kids can work on their school projects," he said. "This has been a real opportunity for those kids who are using the program."

"We have 550 children enrolled and about 250 are there on any given day in the after school program," Stan said. "In some cases they got discouraged at school; for others they have no place to go when classes let out. Too many get involved with gangs or with other activities that aren't productive. All kids—no matter what their background—are welcome. I really believe that Boys & Girls Clubs of America is one of the most significant ways we can impact certain underprivileged kids in our society."

Stan points to former club-member-turned-movie-star Denzel Washington as one famous example of how kids in Boys & Girls Clubs can grow to influence our society. Denzel's mother, Lennis, captures the power of her son's involvement: "I think Denzel learned that men could be gentle, smart, and he could be like that too. It made him a man—that's the beauty of the Club."

Now a national trustee with the Boys & Girls Clubs, Stan is able to reach out all across America, as well as on local levels, influencing the future of thousands of young kids in danger of losing their way.

"I love the quote, 'Ordinary people can do extraordinary things,'" Stan said. "I have learned that we each have certain gifts and everyone has abilities in different areas. Some have gifts of hospitality, some with mentoring, some in service, some in leadership and some in supporting others. I tell my four children that they are special and should really go for life with whatever gifts they have."

Stan and his wife are devoted to kids, whether they are their own or others of God's children. He believes the Boys & Girls Clubs of America are center court in the effort to reach out to the disadvantaged. For these kids, Stan Smith is still serving aces in a "love" game.

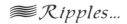 *Ripples...*

Mieasha Hicks

National Youth of the Year, 2004

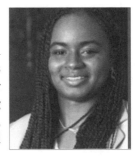

Meet Mieasha Hicks, 18, a member of Boys & Girls Clubs of Toledo, Ohio and Boys & Girls Clubs of America's National Youth of the Year for 2004. The program recognizes outstanding contributions to one's family, school, community, and club, as well as personal challenges and obstacles overcome.

If one word could describe Mieasha, that word would be "survivor." Her parents were 13 and 15 years old when she was born. She was shuffled between households as the family grew. Being the oldest sibling to seven children, Mieasha had no choice but to mature quickly.

Today, she helps her brothers and sisters with their homework and prepares them for tests. She often takes them to the library, the movies, shopping, and out to dinner. Thanks to Mieasha, all of her younger siblings have become honor students.

Mieasha's mother left the state when she was 11, and her father died when she was 12. Despite these traumas, Mieasha's visits to the East Toledo Boys & Girls Clubs gave her a reason to stay positive.

For the following 10 years, the Club has given Mieasha a place to belong. She served as Vice President of the Keystone Club, a group that gave her the opportunity to lead community service projects. She also has learned marketing and retail skills while organizing bake sales and candy sales as fundraisers. Among other activities, Mieasha assisted with Power Hour, her Boys & Girls Club's after-school homework help program.

For winning the National Youth of the Year honor, as well as the Midwest regional title, the Reader's Digest Foundation has awarded Mieasha a combined $15,000 scholarship. With a bright future ahead, she began attending Bowling Green University in 2005, planning to study medicine and science. Thanks to the Boys and Girls Clubs' equipping Mieasha with a positive attitude, emotional stability, a financial scholarship, and hope, her star shines with productive possibilities.

For More Information

Boys & Girls Clubs of America comprises a national network of more than 4,000 neighborhood-based facilities annually serving some 4.8 million young people, primarily from disadvantaged circumstances. They are served by 49,000 trained professional staff and 151,000 volunteers in all 50 states, Puerto Rico and the Virgin Islands, plus nearly 400 domestic and international military bases.

It takes money to run a Boys & Girls Club—on average, about $200 per youth, per year. But consider the alternative: keeping a young adult in jail costs taxpayers anywhere from $25,000 to $75,000 per year. In a recent "Philanthropy 400" report, The Chronicle of Philanthropy ranked Boys & Girls Clubs of America (B&GCA) No. 1 among youth organizations for the 12th consecutive year, and No. 16 among all nonprofit organizations.

Known as "The Positive Place for Kids," the Clubs provide guidance-oriented character development programs on a daily basis for children 6–18 years old, conducted by a full-time professional staff. Key Boys & Girls Club programs, such as Youth of the Year, emphasize character and leadership development, education and career enhancement, health and life skills, the arts, sports and fitness, and recreation.

Millions have benefited from belonging to a Boys & Girls Club since the first Club opened its doors in 1860. Of the participating youth, 80% said Club staff helped them learn right from wrong; 52% said participating in the Club "saved my life!"

Stan Smith. Bill Cosby. Alex Rodriguez. Brad Pitt. Michael Jordan. President Clinton. Jackie Joyner-Kersee. Neil Diamond. Denzel Washington. What do all of these people have in common? They are all alumni of Boys & Girls Clubs of America. While many Club alumni have achieved particular distinction in fields such as entertainment, business, politics and sports, the average alumnus is not famous. Most have achieved success simply by surviving and becoming "out-standing"—getting an education, raising a family, serving their country, pursuing a career or supporting their communities in a variety of ways.

One of the "Best Charities in America" needs you to get involved. Help Boys and Girls. Contact:

Boys & Girls Clubs of America National Headquarters

1275 W. Peachtree Street, NE

Atlanta, Georgia 30309

Phone: (404) 487-5700

E-mail: Info@bgca.org

Website: www.bgca.org

CORPORATE SNAPSHOTS

*"Unless commitment
is made,
there are only promises and hopes...
but no plans."*
—Peter Drucker

*"The more you express gratitude
for what you have,
the more you will have
to express gratitude for."*
—Zig Ziglar

"It's kind of fun to do the impossible."
—Walt Disney

*"The truth of the matter is that there's nothing
you can't accomplish if:
(1) you clearly decide what it is that you're
absolutely committed to achieving,
(2) you're willing to take massive action,
(3) you notice what's working or not, and
(4) you continue to change
your approach until you achieve
what you want, using whatever life gives you along the way."*
—Anthony Robbins

Corporate Snapshots

With American corporate donations to charity increasing by 6% in 2006 to a record $12.72 billion, it can be very inspiring to capture a few snapshots of corporate giants investing in solutions for social challenges. Call it their ROH: Return On Humanity. And it reaches much further than simply writing checks. The volunteer service component of companies all across our country is skyrocketing, even though it does not improve their bottom line. From service companies to retailers and technology innovation companies to manufacturers, corporate America has a momentous and ever-increasing common investment in volunteering, civic responsibility, and active engagement in local, national, and global communities.

A few facts from a 2006 report from the Committee to Encourage Corporate Philanthropy:

♥ More than 85% of all American companies have domestic volunteerism programs in place, and 41% have international volunteerism programs.

♥ Donations by corporations are given 45% in direct cash, 33% in foundation cash, and 22% through products or pro-bono services.

♥ A full 88.6% of corporate giving stays within the United States.

And, according to the Hudson Institute, within three weeks of the devastating earthquake in China's Sichuan province, the United States had pledged $3.1 million in aid, while corporate donations totaled $90 million.

If you look around, you will find thousands of shining beacons of corporate generosity. Here are just a few snapshots from various business sectors:

DISNEY'S UNIQUE Magic ≈ Around the globe, across all its lines of business—including Disney, ABC, and ESPN, The Walt Disney Company uses its unique magic to positively impact children, their communities, and the environment through their Disney VoluntEARS program. Social and community issues have been an important part of the culture of The Walt Disney Company dating back to the Company's founder himself, Walt Disney.

"The greatest moments in life are not concerned with selfish achievements, but rather with the things we do for other people." —Walt Disney

Building on its reputation and using their famous "magic," Disney's "Outreach Mission" is "to brighten the lives of children and families when they need it most." More than 23,000 Disney VoluntEARS around the world invest time and talent year round to enhance their communities.

Granting wishes is also an integral part of Disney's tradition. The Company is the No. 1 granter for the Make-A-Wish Foundation and other similar nonprofits and each year, helps fulfill more than 7,000 Disney related wishes for children with life-threatening conditions. Disney also supports the Starlight/Starbright PC Pals program to bring personal computers into hospitals so children can play games, communicate with other children with similar illnesses, and—most importantly—provide diverting entertainment. Additionally, Disney employees developed and implemented more than 2,200 VoluntEAR projects last year around the world, including redecorating hospital rooms and orphanages, feeding meals to the homeless, planting trees and cleaning up rivers and beaches.

Walt Disney implemented the tradition of corporate giving in the 1930s, when he often visited children in pediatric hospitals in Los Angeles and Disney animators drew for the young patients. Disney's commitment to Boys & Girls Clubs of America also spans more than 50 years, when Walt was made an honorary member of the organization's board of directors. Today 31% of Disney executives serve on boards of nonprofit organizations.

Together with ABC and ESPN, Disney is a beacon of hope for community service, serving through the airwaves to get out positive messages, streaming public service announcements, using celebrities to promote volunteerism, carrying popular pro-service shows like Extreme Makeover: Home Edition and Oprah's Big Give. Disney also has created a special program entitled "Volunteers Across America" that encourages volunteerism.

Examples of Disney senior leadership's commitment to volunteering and community outreach include:

♥ President and CEO Bob Iger led a KaBOOM playground build for his direct reports and another 130 Disney VoluntEARS to benefit more than 300 deserving children in East Los Angeles in December 2007.

♥ ESPN President George Bodenheimer took his leadership teams on a playground build for a Boys & Girls Club on the Gulf Coast.

♥ Andy Mooney, chairman of Disney Consumer Products, has served as the executive champion for the Toys for Tots Foundation drive. He also serves on a board to mentor disadvantaged students. Walt Disney and his animators designed the Foundation's original train logo which is still in use today.

♥ Anne Sweeney, co-chair of Disney Media Networks and president of Disney ABC Television Group, is on the international board of Special Olympics. For the past nine years, Sweeney has served as the executive champion for the Revlon Run Walk for women, joined by 300 Disney VoluntEARS every year, who have raised over $1 million for the cause since the event's inception.

♥ Dick Cook, chairman, The Walt Disney Studios, has served for years as executive champion for the Disney-Salvation Army Thanksgiving dinner benefiting the homeless and working poor.

♥ Ed Grier, president of Disneyland, served as executive champion for Family Volunteer Day in Orange County. He also invited other CEOs and their employees to join Disney VoluntEARS as they packed 14,000-plus food boxes for needy families at a local food bank.

♥ Tom McAlpin, president of Disney Cruise Line, serves on the national board of Make-A-Wish® America.

♥ Jim Fielding, president, Disney Stores Worldwide, serves on the board of the Make-A-Wish Foundation International.

♥ Jeff Hoffman, vice president of Disney Worldwide Outreach, is on the board of Points of Light Institute and HandsOn Network. He also is President of the Volunteer Centers of California and was appointed by Governor Arnold Schwarzenegger to the California Service Corps Commission where he serves as Vice Chair.

Last year, Disney donated more than $177 million in cash and in-kind support to charities around the world, and VoluntEARS contributed more than 466,000 hours of service. Since starting their volunteer program 25 years ago, company employees in more than 42 countries have donated more than 5 million hours to communities in which they live and work. Walt Disney must be smiling! From April 25th 2008 though June 25th 2008, VoluntEARS around the world developed and implemented over 600 projects, impacting over 2 million people.

"Somehow I can't believe that there are any heights that can't be scaled by a man who knows the secrets of making dreams come true. This special secret, it seems to me, can be summarized in four C's. They are curiosity, confidence, courage, and constancy."

—*Walt Disney*

HOME DEPOT Builds ≈ Through their foundation, which was launched in 2002, Home Depot has helped increase access to affordable housing. Their foundation has granted $70 million to nonprofit organizations and has helped develop more than 50,000 houses. In addition, they have supported healthy communities by planting and restoring trees along streets, parks, and in schoolyards, helping build and refurbish community play spaces, and doing what they can to revitalize school facilities.

Through Team Depot, employees work side by side to create meaningful lifelong relationships with their neighbors, volunteering professional expertise and helping hands.

In 2007, Home Depot Foundation supported the production of 12,223 affordable housing units, planted or restored more than 310,000 community trees, completed a three-year, $25 million agreement with KaBOOM! to create and refurbish 1,000 play spaces in 1,000 days, built

130 playgrounds, made grants totaling almost $40 million to more than 1,350 nonprofits, awarded more than $1.5 million to 520 nonprofits, and matched more than $4.6 million in charitable contributions made by Home Depot associates. Employees themselves donated more than 530,000 hours of volunteer service.

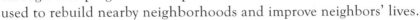

The green in Home Depot's logo might reflect The Framing Hope Program, which helps communities and improves the environment. Products donated through this program are kept out of landfills and used to rebuild nearby neighborhoods and improve neighbors' lives.

Home Depot exemplifies building hope through commitment.

CHICK-FIL-A's Tender Heart ≈ Chick-fil-A Founder Truett Cathy first opened his heart and home to children more than 30 years ago. Since then, his desire to inspire young people has continued to grow. Driven by his interest in the growth and education of young people, Truett and his wife, Jeannette, established the WinShape Foundation in 1984 with one goal: to help "shape winners."

The foundation supports a variety of programs, including a long-term foster care program, a summer camp for nearly 1,800 kids each year, marriage enrichment retreats, and a co-op scholarship program in conjunction with Berry College, based in Rome, Georgia.

WinShape Foundation expanded in 1987 with the addition of WinShape Homes to provide foster care to children who need a loving, nurturing, stable, secure family environment in which to grow. There are currently 11 homes—eight in Georgia, one in Alabama, and two in Tennessee.

Each home is licensed to accommodate up to 12 children and employs a set of full-time house parents. WinShape Homes' foster care program is unique in several ways. They give large sibling groups an opportunity to remain together as a family, rather than being separated, a frequent occurrence when large families enter foster care. The homes also encourage the children's participation in extra-curricular activities and provide services to meet the children's physical, spiritual, and emotional needs. WinShape Homes is unique in its encouragement and provision of the pursuit of a college or technical degree for each child.

WinShape International is WinShape Foundation's newest program, started in 2005, to equip motivated young adults to become Christian leaders within their own cultures. Their mission is to mobilize leaders to transform young people and communities around the world. Together they pursue projects that are sustainable, reproducible, measurable and beneficial over a long period of time.

Cathy's original vision to encourage young people to be "winners and leaders" has steadily grown over the past 24 years and no doubt will continue to expand, pursuing WinShapes' mission of shaping individuals to be winners. Truett, you're a gold medal winner!

> *"Nearly every moment of every day we have the opportunity to give something to someone else—our time, our love, our resources. I have always found more joy in giving when I did not expect anything in return."* —S. Truett Cathy

GENERAL ELECTRIC's (GE) Imagination at Work ≈ Total giving for the GE Foundation in 2006 was more than $200 million, including a $100 million investment to improve student achievement and increase college-readiness across targeted school districts – but that doesn't begin to tell the story of their involvement.

With 350,000 employees worldwide, GE is committed to encouraging service and involvement, both financially and personally. They have a matching grant program for employees and retirees, and everyone is encouraged to donate to a favorite cause and have their dollars multiplied for good. GE also encourages active volunteerism by their employees in the areas of education, environment, and community development in over 140 locations around the world. In 2007, GE employees and retirees combined volunteered more than 1 million hours of community service.

Excellence in education is a primary focus of GE's foundation. They partner with schools and organizations to develop high-impact programs, both in America and abroad. GE supports scholarships that encourage students from under-represented or disadvantaged backgrounds to pursue a higher education degree, with a special emphasis on studies in science, engineering, technology, or business. Globally, GE emphasizes early education preparedness, especially in China, India, and Mexico.

Through hands-on commitment in more than 38 countries and grants made possible through the donations of the GE family, they have supported senior centers, children with autism, literacy for low-income communities, neglected urban spaces, and many other worthy programs.

Their disaster relief fund helps rebuild lives and communities devastated by natural tragedies. A few examples of GE goodwill:

♥ With thousands of brushes, gallons of paint and immeasurable goodwill, employees made the first-ever Planet PaintFest program the largest and most comprehensive volunteer effort in GE volunteer history. It has transformed hundreds of the world's hospitals into more colorful environments for healing.

♥ In Cincinnati, Ohio, more than 1,600 GE volunteers participate in a cluster of education projects focused on strategic partnerships with some very challenged inner-city schools. Supported by the GE Foundation Developing Futures in Education program, "Mission Possible" has donated more than 11,000 volunteer hours annually to educational initiatives that include mentoring, tutoring, homework help, exploring engineering, and computer lab. College-bound rates increased from 8% to more than 60% and proficiency scores, attendance, passing, and graduation rates rose.

♥ São Paolo now has an unusual soap factory with the assistance of a GE Volunteers Foundation grant. The factory recycles used, donated cooking oil, which is screened and mixed with other products and transformed into ecologic soap. The factory facility also maintains daycare centers and provides classes in academic subjects, leisure activities and dance. Today, the factory has eight employees, most of them parents of the children served by the daycare centers. This work not only creates income and sustainability, but also protects the environment.

♥ GE's Developing Health Globally initiative (formerly called Africa Project) began in 2004 with a $20-million product donation commitment in rural African communities, and has since expanded to a five-year, $30-million program. It is designed to improve healthcare delivery in rural African and Latin American communities, and ultimately other regions of the world. In Ghana, hospital outpatient visits to rural district hospitals have increased by as much as 99% over a one-year period, and referral cases have declined by as much as 60% in the same time period. Hospital births and equipment utilization have also increased, indicating an increase in community confidence and trust in the healthcare system and public healthcare facilities.

The GE Foundation supports the educational programming of Junior Achievement in schools worldwide. JA seeks to inspire young people to succeed in a global economy by providing K–12 curriculum that teaches free enterprise, business, economics, ethics, citizenship, and financial literacy.

GE's commitment to making a difference in the world is absolutely electric!

COSTCO Connects ≈ Costco and Newman's Own®. The idea to co-brand Newman's Own® grape juice initially came as a shock to Tim Rose, Costco's senior vice-president of foods and sundries, but it was an offer he couldn't refuse. In creating Kirkland Signature—Newman's Own Grape Juice, a new model for corporate philanthropy was born. Newman's Own and Costco split the profits from their joint venture, with Costco donating 100 percent of its gross profits to the Children's Miracle Network, and Newman's Own funneling its share to any of the 30 charities it supports. With this innovative concept, everyone wins—especially the kids who need it most.

About two years ago, as his teenage son was fighting cancer, Tim saw a video about Newman's Hole in the Wall Gang Camps for children stricken with serious illnesses. He was inspired to bring a similar camp to the Pacific Northwest, home to Costco's headquarters.

Camp Korey is named after Tim's 18-year-old son, whose life was cut short in 2004 by osteo sarcoma, a bone cancer. Located in Redmond, Washington, this camp will be a special spot where seriously ill children can safely forget about the limitations of their ailments. Camp Korey, scheduled to open in 2008, will be an affiliate of the Hole in the Wall Gang Camps, founded by Paul Newman in 1988. Currently ten such camps exist worldwide, serving thousands of kids a year. All children who attend the camps, no matter their illnesses or capacity, can fully participate in every activity because liberating full-access components are built into camp facilities. All campers attend free of charge, thanks to generous contributions from individuals, corporations, and foundations.

At Tim's suggestion, Costco again partnered with Newman's Own to create a breakfast cereal, Newman's Own Hole in the Wall Cereal, which is sold exclusively in Costco stores. Once again, with 100% of the profits from the sale of the cereal donated to the camps and to children's hospitals, Costco and Newman's Own are helping the kids who need it most.

"Nothing makes us happier than sending checks out to help children, whether it is through hospitals, camps or scholarships," Tim said. "It just tickles us pink."

Whether pink or red, Costco and Newman's Own together are forming rainbows of corporate love to kids who need them most.

BEN & JERRY'S is Sweet ≈ As a corporation, Ben & Jerry's Homemade Inc. has been churning out blissful dollops of ice cream since 1978, when the two young entrepreneurs made a $12,000 investment ($4,000 of it was borrowed) and opened their first homemade ice cream scoop shop in a renovated gas station in Burlington, Vermont. From the beginning, the two decided to also churn out good will and give back to their community. Their altruism stemmed from the belief co-founders Ben Cohen and Jerry Greenfield shared that businesses have a responsibility for community involvement. In 1985, the founders created the Ben & Jerry's Foundation and makes grants to grassroots organizations in the United States that address social or environmental problems.

In Vermont, where the company is based, Ben & Jerry's has reached out to the DREAM program, a Vermont AmeriCorps state program. Working through the DREAM Program, families and college students mentor children from affordable-housing neighborhoods to recognize their options, make informed decisions, and achieve their dreams.

In May 2005, 65 employees from Ben & Jerry's South Burlington corporate offices spent a day at Camp DREAM, a residential summer camp where participants eight years of age and older can spend a week at summer camp for free. During that day of service, employees helped build a low ropes course, construct a canoe rack, and break ground for an organic garden. The energy of that day set the tone for a new tradition of camp days.

When DREAM became an AmeriCorps program in 2007 and needed office space, Ben & Jerry's stepped in to provide rooms in their corporate headquarters. The company welcomed the DREAM staff to the building, offered organizational advice, and donated printing to DREAM's annual appeal. And to sweeten the relationship, DREAM staff offer taste tips on ice cream products.

That's cool!

AT&T Foundation's Calling ≈ In reaction to the fact that nearly one-third of U.S. high school students are dropping out of high school, AT&T launched AT&T Aspire, a $100 million philanthropic program to help strengthen student success and workforce readiness.

Announced in April 2008, Aspire supports the work of the education community to help kids succeed in school and realize the connection between education and their best possible future.

The program will work to address this issue by:

♥ Providing $100 million in grants to schools and nonprofits with proven success in helping students stay in school and prepare for college or the workforce.

♥ Utilizing the nation's largest company-sponsored volunteer organization, the AT&T Pioneers, and working with Junior Achievement, providing 100,000 students with the opportunity to shadow AT&T employees companywide, and see firsthand the kinds of skills they'll need to be successful in the workplace.

♥ Helping to fund 100 community dropout prevention summits, which are being organized by America's Promise Alliance across all 50 states to engage education experts and community leaders around the crisis and ways to address it.

♥ In partnership with America's Promise, AT&T is commissioning major national research by John Bridgeland, following on his landmark study "The Silent Epidemic." This new research will garner the practitioner perspective (teachers, principals, superintendents, and school board members) on the root causes and most effective solutions to address the dropout crisis.

"One-third of U.S. students dropping out equates to one student every 26 seconds, and as a corporate citizen, AT&T is concerned about this loss of human potential," said Laura Sanford, president of the AT&T Foundation. "We wanted to support the great and much needed work already underway to address this issue while adding our own touch."

Dropouts are far more likely than high school graduates to be unemployed, living in poverty, in poor health, or in prison. As a major U.S. corporation, the company is also concerned how the dropout issue affects America's ability to compete in the global economy. Students unprepared to enter college cost the U.S. economy more than $3.7 billion annually in lost earnings and remedial education costs.

The AT&T Aspire program is AT&T's most significant education initiative to date, and one of the largest ever corporate commitments to address the specific issues of high school success and workforce readiness.

"Investing in a well-educated workforce may be the single most important thing we can do to help America remain the leader in a digital, global economy, while at the same time ensuring a brighter future for our children," Sanford remarked. "AT&T is proud to be a part of this investment."

FERGUSON's Plumbing Possibilities ≈ Headquartered in Newport News, Virginia, Ferguson is the country's largest wholesale distributor of plumbing supplies: pipes, valves and fittings; heating and cooling equipment; waterworks; bathrooms and appliances, etc. With sales of $11 billion, their 1,400 service centers are located in all 50 states, Puerto Rico, Mexico and the Caribbean. Philanthropically working with 22,000 associates, Ferguson helps achieve affordable housing by supporting Habitat for Humanity with toilets and supplies, as well as lots of volunteer time for home builds. Their associates also raise money for cancer research, and donate to support civic, educational, and environmental causes.

Educationally, Ferguson supports the Boys and Girls Club and many local projects. Ferguson financially sponsors K.I.C.K., Kids Involved in Community Kindness, which is a service-learning curriculum, developed by Alternatives, Inc., a nationally recognized nonprofit youth development organization based near Ferguson's corporate headquarters. K.I.C.K. gives young people the opportunity to discover the joy and satisfaction of service to others. With the K.I.C.K. curriculum, even the newest service-learning practitioner can take young people through the steps of a quality educational project by simply following their service curriculum

In their headquarters community of Hampton Roads, Virginia, Ferguson supports Achievable Dream. Achievable Dream has been recognized as a ground-breaking effort to turn the tide of inner city underperformance in education. Ferguson has also joined forces with New Horizons Regional Educational Center to make and distribute a unique learning tool for elementary students. "Fun Phones," consisting of plastic pipes fitted together in the shape of a traditional phone handle, amplifies sound so users can hear themselves more clearly than by reading out loud. Students having difficulty with pronunciation can listen in a more perceptible way to their speech pattern—even in a crowded classroom. These phones increase reading comprehension, help students focus on their pronunciation, and improve attention and memory.

"Ferguson is honored to donate material to support the Fun Phone project," said John Stegeman, president and chief executive officer for Ferguson. "This unique partnership utilizes one of Ferguson's most popular products, PVC pipe, to further our organization's unwavering commitment to support the communities in which we do business and lend a helping hand to children."

Ferguson is flush with justified pride in their effort to help build communities.

PFIZER's Good Medicine ≈ Pfizer Incorporated topped the list of the largest corporate givers in 2006 with $1.7 billion donated in both cash and products, according to *The Chronicle of Philanthropy*. This New York corporation strives to improve the health of people all over the world, investing the full range of their resources–people, skills, expertise, and funding–to broaden access to medicines and strengthen healthcare delivery for under-served populations. To accomplish this goal, Pfizer partners with non-governmental organizations, governments, and private-sector partners through long-term, sustainable programs to achieve global health outcomes.

While Pfizer is mobilized globally to combat major killers like malaria and HIV/AIDS, the company also initiated a long-term program in 1998 to eliminate trachoma, the world's leading cause of preventable blindness. Partnering with the World Health Organization (WHO), Gates Foundation, Lions, USAID, and the Edna McConnell Clark Foundation, among others, and through the International Trachoma Initiative, Pfizer has distributed more than 77 million treatments of their Zithromax® drug in 16 countries. Are they making a difference? Ask people in Morocco, who live in the first country to complete the campaign for trachoma control (in 2006). Morocco is working toward WHO certification now that trachoma has been eliminated as a public health problem.

Pfizer has strong medicine for global health issues!

And just to salute charitable giving through a few other corporations in 2006, according to the Chronicles of Philanthropy's 2007 study:

♥ Wal-Mart gave a total of $264 million, the largest percentage of all-cash giving.

♥ Microsoft, with the largest foundation in the world, gave $436 million.

♥ Merck, the pharmaceutical giant, gave $826 million in cash and product.

While we live in a country where every contribution counts, the compassion and giving of American corporations is astounding. We live in a land of benevolent giants!

SALUTE TO
SPORTS PASSIONARIES

"The difference between the impossible
and the possible
lies in a person's determination."
　　　　　　—Tommy Casorda

"It is time for us all to stand and cheer
for the doer, the achiever—
the one who recognizes the challenge
and does something about it."
　　　　　　—Vince Combardi

"Reach down and lift others up.
It's the best exercise you can get."
　　　　　　—Anonymous

"Do not let what you cannot do
interfere with what you can do."
　　　　　　—John Wooden

Snapshots of Sports Passionaries

Sports Champions are hailed as heroes and rightfully crowned for their prowess and victories. Many sports figures are real heroes off the fields of play, championing people in need whose plight has touched their hearts. Their trophy is the smile of one person touched, a wrong righted, a soul saved. They move the ball forward, focused on the goal of helping others find success. They are experts on how to rally around a loss. Consider the real victories in a few snapshot samples of sports passionaries.

Alex Smith

49ers Quarterback

The Alex Smith Foundation

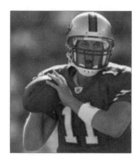

Putting Foster Kids in the End Zone

"Why does our society spend billions of dollars on foster children, only to abandon these kids when they're on the verge of becoming adults? It seems like we're dropping the ball at the goal line."

—Alex Smith

When Alex Smith became the No. 1 pick in the 2005 NFL draft, he knew he wanted to help his community in a significant way. Instead of just writing checks, he wanted to do something that would directly affect lives.

Alex was invited one day to meet a champion eight-man football team from a residential San Diego high school for foster children. He sensed an opportunity to start helping others.

"I went and met with some of the teens there and was able to donate shoes for every kid in the school," Alex said. "As I talked to them and heard their stories, it hit me: I'm not that far removed from them in age, and I couldn't imagine what it would be like to live without any support."

That was the beginning of a continuing effort to help San Francisco Bay Area foster children who have not been given the tools necessary to succeed in school and life. When a foster child reaches age 18, they are "emancipated" and turned loose on their own. Without any support, they face enormous hurdles.

Alex can rattle off the statistics from memory: In the state of California, within 18 months of emancipation, more than 60% of former foster youths are unemployed. More than 25% experience homelessness at least once after leaving foster care. And within two years, 25% will be in prison. "It's something I'm striving to change," Alex said. "It's something we need to change."

At a child welfare conference, Alex met Antwone Fisher, who was born in prison and spent 18 years in the foster care system. On his 18th birthday, his social worker took him to a men's shelter. "He gave me $70 and told me I was on my own," Antwone said. "But it was too dangerous for me to live at the shelter."

Homeless on the streets of Cleveland, Ohio, Antwone slept in storefronts and sometimes in the snow. He escaped his situation by joining the United States Navy, serving his country for 11 years. Afterward, he moved to California and became an author and playwright.

As Alex and Antwone talked, an idea was born: the Alex Smith Foundation, dedicated to raising awareness about the alarming statistics of young people transitioned out of foster care. "I had never heard of anyone caring about foster kids," Antwone said. "What Alex is trying to do is one of the most important things you can do for a foster kid. Like myself, if you don't have anything or anybody and you find there is somebody out there who cares, that means a lot."

The Alex Smith Foundation provides money for existing transitional programs and works to create new avenues to provide mentoring, job training, and continuing education for 4,000 youth who transition out of California's foster care system each year. The goal is to ensure that they will not be abandoned, as Antwone Fisher was years ago.

"Antwone has such an amazing story," Alex said. "I asked him to help me out on my endeavor. I want to be successful with this."

"When I went off to college, my parents drove me there, bought me a computer, and gave me money for anything I needed to succeed in school," Alex said. "I've got a huge support system and I relied on them so much. I would not be who I am today without that support team. There are kids who are abandoned, and it's tragic that they've been left without anyone. We can do better."

Last year, Alex partnered with San Diego State University to create a Guardian Scholars Program, which seeks to help foster youths make the transition to adulthood. The program provides high school graduates with five-year scholarships to SDSU, where they will receive year-round housing and one-on-one guidance.

The San Diego State Guardian Scholars program became the 22nd in a network of California campuses. More than 200 former foster youth are now in college under this program and they have a graduation rate of 70 percent, which is higher than for regular students.

San Francisco Mayor Gavin Newsom, whose own family has fostered children, praises Smith's work: "I care deeply about this because I see the impact families have in changing peoples' lives. My family wasn't successful. We had three foster youth, and two of them landed in San Quentin. We've got to be there when they are emancipated. We've got to step up and do what's right."

"The spirit of Alex's foundation is changing lives," concludes Mayor Newsom. "There's nothing you look back on in your life with more pride than having an impact on changing someone's life in a positive way."

For More Information

Get off the sidelines and help carry the ball over the goal line for foster kids transitioning. Contact:

The Alex Smith Foundation

Phone: (619) 980-3469

Website: alexsmithfoundation.org

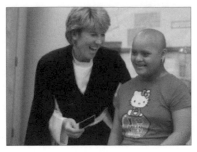

Andrea Jaeger
Tennis Champion

Silver Lining Camps

Serving Up a Love Game

It's hard to picture Sister Andrea, now an Episcopalian Nun in a flowing black habit, having worn a short tennis skirt. But in 1979 as Andrea Jaeger—a 14-year-old, pigtailed tennis phenom with braces—she became a successful professional tennis player.

Andrea beat some of the best tennis players in the world, from Billie Jean King to Chris Evert to Martina Navratilova. At 16, she ranked second in the world, winning the French Open on her birthday. At 19 though, she was done—forced from the game by a severe shoulder injury that would require seven surgeries and three years to repair.

What's important in the life of Andrea Jaeger is what happened to her between the pigtails and the nun's habit.

Andrea has devoted the past 20 years to healing the broken hearts of children who are fighting cancer. "Nobody knows if you have tomorrow," Andrea said. "I want them to have life while they're alive, to be in a place where nobody isolates them because they are different."

The youth outreach started in 1990, when Andrea and humanitarian businesswoman Heidi Bookout teamed up to form Silver Lining Foundation, now called Little Star Foundation, a nonprofit program for children suffering from cancer and other diseases. Andrea used her $1.4 million in tennis earnings as seed money as they set out to change the world. The Foundation's programs have since reached thousands of children stricken by disease, neglect, and poverty. Outreach efforts include distributing medical supplies, equipment, food, clothing, and educational materials worldwide.

In 1999, construction of their Silver Lining Ranch was completed in Aspen, Colorado on 10 acres donated by a local couple. Businessman Ted Forstmann made a $1.7 million down payment toward the

18,000-square-foot, $6 million complex. Other donations—many from tennis celebrities—followed.

Jaeger and her ranch colleagues bring young cancer patients together for white-water rafting, horseback riding, skiing, canoeing, and laughter. It's a week away from hospitals and painful tests. Twenty youngsters from around the country, usually between ages 9 and 17, come for a week at a time. The campers are chosen because they are well enough for the adventure, but their prognoses are poor. Of the 12 Chicago youngsters in Andrea's first session a decade ago, only one is still alive—but she is a mother.

Andrea said: "The whole mission of the Foundation is to create opportunities for children with cancer and other life-threatening diseases to improve their lives."

Spirits are lifted with the help of celebrities like John McEnroe, Andre Agassi, Pete Sampras, Paul Newman, Valerie Bertinelli and David Robinson. Kevin Costner takes children fishing at his nearby ranch. Cindy Crawford, who lost a brother to leukemia, helps children accept how cancer has changed their appearance. "Andrea does this for all the right reasons and it shines through her actions," Cindy said. "She is completely devoted to helping others."

The Foundation must raise $4.3 million each year. Andrea also sponsors reunions, family retreats, college scholarships, internships, and for children who can't travel, programs that come to them.

Little Star Foundation also helps kids recovering from abuse, war, and other traumatic circumstances. Close friend and former rival Billie Jean King said: "Andrea has done so much good for so many others since leaving tennis, and her journey continues today."

Andrea said that when she hears stories of children dying from cancer, her heart is "ripped into a million pieces."

"You watch these kids and they don't know whether the next day is going to be their last, and yet they bring joy, love, and laughter," Andrea said. "You get thoughts of what they go through, and you get caught up in the energy and excitement of helping. That's what I hold on to."

Andrea adds: "I believe in the philosophy of one child at a time. If you can make a child smile or laugh, your place in the world has been preserved. You carry a lot of what the kids bring and when you see their strength, their character, the hope in their eyes and in their heart, it gets you through the darkest hours you could ever have."

"She follows her heart," said Andrea's sister, Suzanne. "Andrea has always followed her heart. Many people don't have the strength to do that."

And as Sister Andrea, she is still following her heart, living a life to serve God and help children.

For More Information

Helping kids in crisis is a smashing love game. Place the ball in Andrea's court and contact:

Little Star Foundation
256 Rancho Milagro Way
Hesperus, Colorado 81326
Phone (800) 543-6565
E-mail: info@littlestar.org
Website: www.littlestar.org

*"The beauty of empowering others
is that your own power
is not diminished in the process."
—Barbara Colorose*

Dick Vitale
Basketball: Sportscaster

The V Foundation

Fighting Cancer, Helping Kids

"It's Awesome, Baby! I'm living the American dream. I learned from my mom and dad, who didn't have a formal education but had doctorates of love."

—Dick Vitale

Dick "Dickie V" Vitale coached the National Basketball Association's Detroit Pistons for one season before being fired. While waiting for another coaching job, he gave analysis and color coverage for the first college basketball game to be televised on a new sports network, ESPN. That was 30 years ago. Vitale never made it back to coaching. Instead he became a popular mainstay at ESPN, where he now has called more than 1,000 games.

Dick is under contract with ESPN through 2013. On the air, he is recognized for his thorough knowledge of the game, his preparation, and an enthusiastic, passionate style that is sometimes controversial but never boring. Then there are his catchphrases: "Awesome, baby!", "Get a TO!" (time-out), "PTP'er" (prime-time player), and "diaper dandy" (freshman talent).

"People told me that if you gave 110 percent all the time, many beautiful things will happen," Dick said. "I may not always be right, but no one can ever accuse me of not having a genuine love and passion for whatever I do."

Dick's enthusiasm carries over to his philanthropy. He and his wife, Lorraine, spend the off-season in Sarasota, Florida, where for many years he has supported the local Boys & Girls Club. His annual banquet has raised more than $1 million for a new physical education and health training center. "This is a home away from home for many youngsters who come from single-parent and economically disadvantaged environments," Dick said. "Kids learn the value of education and the dangers of drugs and alcohol. They enjoy crafts, computers, and sports." Each Christmas, the Vitale family opens their home to needy children from the Boys and Girls Club for dinner and gifts.

Dick also is an enthusiastic and passionate worker for The V Foundation, formed in honor of former North Carolina State men's basketball coach Jimmy Valvano. Vitale and Valvano (or Dick and Jimmy) worked together at ESPN, and the two "Vs" once appeared together in a comedy sketch on the Bill Cosby show. Valvano died of cancer in 1993 at the age of 47. Since it was launched, The V Foundation has raised more than $30 million and awarded more than 200 research grants to fight this disease.

"I remember when Jimmy broke the news of his disease to me, how we both wept on the phone," Dick recalled. "He wasn't going to be able to fulfill many of the special dreams he had that involved his wife, Pam, and their beautiful children. Near the end, Jim gathered his closest friends and told us of his desire to beat cancer: 'We can beat this disease if you don't forget me, and raise millions and millions of dollars.'"

As a board member for The V Foundation since its beginning, Dick keeps the pledge he made to his former colleague by holding an annual celebrity fund-raiser gala, bringing in more than $1 million a year for cancer research grants. Celebrities from every sport and ESPN attend and help fill the coffers for the fight against cancer.

Dick got a scare himself in late 2007 when doctors discovered and removed ulcerated lesions from his left vocal cord. They were non-cancerous, but the healing required Dick to not speak for nearly a month. About this time, five-year-old Payton Wright, a friend of Dick's, died of a rare form of brain cancer.

Once he was cleared to speak again, Dick announced a personal war on children's cancer. "I am on a mission," he wrote, describing a plan to raise $1 million in 2008 for the Payton Wright Research Grant to fight cancer in children. "I am driven to help people battle that disease."

"I hope I inspire others to give back and get involved," Dick said. "People who are fortunate enough to make it in life, I hope, will be willing to share some time with youngsters. The smiles on the faces of these little ones are the best present of all."

┌─ **For More Information** ─────────────────────┐

Leave a legacy of hope for cancer victims in memory of coaching legend Jimmy Valvano with education, research, and advocacy on cancer issues:

The V Foundation for Cancer Research

106 Towerview Court

Cary, North Carolina 27513

Website: www.jimmyv.org
└──┘

Tiger Woods
Golf Pro
Start Something

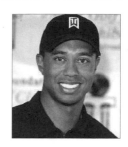

Tiger Tees up for Kids

"I challenge you. I dare you. I challenge you to be a winner in whatever you choose to do, whatever you care about. I challenge you to make a difference in the world, to reach higher and farther than you ever imagined."

—Tiger Woods to the youth of America

On the golf course, Eldrick "Tiger" Woods has done just about everything a golfer could do. At age two, he putted on television with Bob Hope; he scored his first hole in one at age eight—and 17 more since! He has captured 87 tournament wins, 65 of those on the PGA Tour, including the four Majors that make up golf's "Grand Slam." He earns about $100 million a year in winnings and endorsements.

Golf is Tiger's profession, but educating kids is his passion. "Without a doubt," he said, "when I retire from golf, that's all I'm going to do." Tiger Woods and his late father, Earl, a former Green Beret officer who served two tours of duty in Vietnam, brought their family motto of "caring and sharing" to life in 1996 when Tiger Woods Foundation was established. The foundation already has inspired and supported more than 10 million boys and girls. Through its work, Tiger passes on his family values of integrity, honesty, discipline, and fun to a new generation.

Since 1996, Tiger Woods Foundation has invested in communities through more than $30 million in grants to local youth programs. And in 2001, it teamed up with Target Corporation to create "Start Something," an educational program for kids eight to 17. More than 5 million youngsters have enrolled in the free program which focuses on character education, volunteer service, and career exploration. Through participation in Start Something, youth set their sights on a specific personal goal and develop an action plan to achieve it. They also learn to give back to their community and explore careers that match their interests.

Tiger Woods Foundation's most visible project is the Tiger Woods Learning Center, a $25 million project that opened in 2006 in Anaheim, California. This 35,000-square-foot educational facility provides youth with an enrichment program to improve individual aptitude in reading, math, science, language arts, and technology. More than 15,000 students in the Orange County area of Los Angeles use the day program for grades four through six or the after-school program for grades seven through 12. They develop personal accountability, independence, and resilience—leading to greater knowledge of career choices and an interest in attending college. There also are summer and weekend programs, as well as community outreach initiatives including online classes. And yes, there is a golf teaching area too!

Tiger and his foundation also provide university scholarships, maintain an association with Target House, the family accommodations apartments at St. Jude Hospital in Memphis, Tennessee, and host junior golf clinics. Tiger is a favorite of the youngsters taking part in the Make-A-Wish program for seriously ill children. At every junior golf clinic, Tiger spends personal time with one or more Make-A-Wish children.

"I was raised in a household in which, if I did not have my homework done, I could not go play with my friends," Tiger said. "It was always school first; the No. 1 priority in my family." Tiger Woods believes being a good role model is even more important than golf but, through golf, he can positively influence others.

And that's what drives Tiger Woods.

(Story adapted from Tiger Woods web site at tigerwoods.com)

Ripples from
Roberto Clemente
Baseball Legend

Steve Pindar and Roberto's Kids

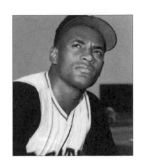

Keeping a Legacy Alive

"We need to show love and to love, not only our kids and our family as a whole but also our neighbors. We're all brothers and sisters, and we must give one another a helping hand when it is needed."

—Roberto Clemente

Roberto Clemente died on New Year's Eve in 1972 when his airplane carrying food and medical supplies to Nicaragua in the wake of a devastating earthquake crashed in the ocean off Puerto Rico shortly after takeoff. His body was never found. During his 17 seasons with baseball's Pittsburgh Pirates, Clemente won four National League Batting Championships, 12 Gold Glove Awards for fielding ability, and played in a dozen All-Star games as well as two World Series championships. He had exactly 3,000 hits when his life ended at age 38.

Major League Baseball honored Clemente's career and service to others by electing him to the National Baseball Hall of Fame without the mandatory five-year waiting period—the first Latino to receive that prestigious award. MLB also created the annual Roberto Clemente Award, presented each year to an active baseball player who best represents his humanitarian work. Thirty years after Roberto's death, President George W. Bush presented his family with the Presidential Medal of Freedom, the highest civilian award in America.

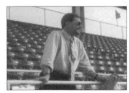

Roberto's name and service legacy are honored today in a special way—through "Roberto's Kids"—a private effort begun by Steve Pindar. Collecting new and "gently worn" baseball equipment, the organization distributes the gear to disadvantaged children in the Dominican Republic and Puerto Rico. One recent shipment contained more than 30,000 items collected from organizations, teams, retail stores, and individuals across 26 states in the United States and three provinces in Canada.

Away from Roberto's Kids, Steve works in VolunTourism through his family's Christian-based mission effort in New York, supporting developing countries in the areas of health, education, and sports. "My baseball program started as a small project in my garage," Steve said. "At the end of the 1999 season, our local Little League had some equipment and uniforms it wasn't going to use again, and I had a family trip planned to the Dominican Republic. So several duffel bags went in with our luggage." When word got around, the project overflowed the garage, spilled into the basement, and took over the Pindars' front porch. Roberto's Kids was born.

The program is endorsed by the Baseball Hall of Fame and Clemente's family. Roberto's youngest son, Luis, notes: "Roberto's Kids has brought joy to those who don't always get the opportunities. It is truly making a difference by inspiring so many others. It follows the Clemente tradition of giving and caring for others."

Steve said, "People, by nature, want to help others. When someone hears about Roberto's Kids, they know we have something important for them to do. We allow them to reach out, be an answer to someone's plea, and find their own passion." He takes special pride watching a team of Dominican youngsters take the field wearing uniforms for the first time. "Many of these kids have never worn shoes before while running the bases," notes Steve.

"When one has the courage to live their life in service to others, you ignite a purpose and everything you touch will be forever changed," Steve adds. "My torch is Roberto's Kids. It is the candle to my soul that I hold out to the world every day. That quiet, inviting flicker is a gentle reminder to live life with passion, making a difference in the lives of others on purpose. There is only enough light to take your journey step-by-step, but that is all any of us really needs."

Roberto Clemente would agree.

Batter-up, and hit a homerun for kids. Connect for the children of the Dominican Republic and contact:

Roberto's Kids

55 Union Street

Oneonta, New York 13820

Phone: (607) 432-7440

Website: www.robertos-kids.org

*"If you think you're
        too small to have an impact,
   try going to bed with a mosquito."*
                    —Anita Roddick

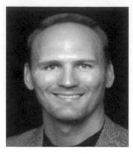

Donnie Dee
National Football League

Fellowship of Christian Athletes

Huddling with Kids for Christ and Sport

"I've been given a gift, and now I want to honor God who gave me that gift. FCA first communicated the Gospel truth to me. I will always be grateful. I will always serve this ministry—not out of obligation or job description—but out of a grateful heart."
—Donnie Dee

It takes a big man to play the position of tight end in the National Football League (NFL). And it takes a huge heart to reach out to tens of thousands of kids struggling to find values and meaning in drug-infested, gang-controlled, hope-deprived inner-city neighborhoods.

Donnie Dee meets both standards. At 6'5" and 250 pounds, he was an imposing force for nearly three seasons with the Indianapolis Colts and the Seattle Seahawks football teams. In 1997, he was asked to work as director for the sprawling Southern California region of a Christian youth outreach he dearly loved, the Fellowship of Christian Athletes (FCA). He and his family loved living in Colorado and hadn't heard anything good about Southern California, but knew this huge region had no FCA staff, office or even a board of directors. Determined, Donnie and his wife Jackie took their young children and made the move thinking of this as a short-term mission that might last a few years.

Formed in 1954, FCA is the largest Christian sports organization in America. It serves local communities by equipping, empowering, and encouraging people to make a difference for Christ. FCA operates across America based on "huddles"—a program at a middle school, high school, or college where one or more FCA members, usually coaches, meet regularly with young school athletes and students.

Donnie notes FCA's explosive growth in recent years: "Nationally, we have about 7,500 huddles that meet weekly or every two weeks. We ran 160 different camps last year with more than 10,000 coaches and athletes attending. We have thousands and thousands of volunteers. We have outreach events with the Super Bowl, college basketball's Final Four, the baseball and hockey All-Star Games, and all the major football bowl games. We are expanding in urban ministry and international events."

Ten years after Donnie's move to Southern California in 1997, the skills he learned from football and life—focus, drive, persistence and leadership—have helped create an explosion of FCA growth for kids. From 10 huddles, there are more than 215 groups that meet weekly on campuses from San Diego to San Luis Obispo. With 30 on staff, there will be 700 high school students who will attend camp in the summer. Seventy to 80 community leaders serve on his FCA boards throughout the region. "Even though the move from Colorado was uncertain and scary, we know God asked Jackie and I to give up something good for something better. It's been really exciting to see what God has done and what He had in mind," Donnie notes. "With about 4 million kids and 1,200 school campuses in Southern California, we still have our work cut out for us."

Professionals in various fields of athletics have come alongside Donnie to build the program, including tennis champ Michael Chang, Miami Dolphins coach Cam Cameron, NFL star Vince Evans, British Open champion, Tom Lehmen, and basketball great A. C. Green. Donnie envisions a great future for FCA. "God is using coaches to have an impact on kids, and I see great opportunities for that in the future," Donnie shares. "God willing, FCA will continue to shape the lives of young athletes for years to come."

Donnie fondly recalls a recent camp setting where, one by one, the campers—300 in all—unexpectedly got out of their seats and came forward to join the band onstage. "I got a little picture of heaven in my mind," Donnie said. "It was black, white, Latino, Samoan, Asian, big kid, little kid, football players, skateboarders, tennis players. They were all at the front of this church with their arms around one another, singing "God of Wonders ... You are holy, You are holy, You are holy."

For More Information

Get in world-class shape: practice, practice, practice loving kids. Connect with FCA:

FCA World Headquarters
8701 Leeds Road
Kansas City, Misssori 64129
Phone: (800) 289-0909
E-mail: fca@fca.org
Website: www.fca.org

Southern California FCA
PO Box 2196
Vista, California 92085
Phone: (760) 720-0341
Website: www.socalfca.org

*"I run the first half of the race
as fast as I can
and then with God's help
I run the second half even faster."*
—Eric Liddell

Lance Armstrong
Champion Bicyclist

Live Strong

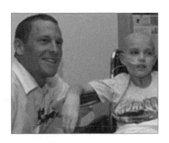

Cancer survivors: Take Charge of Your Life

"October 2, 1996. The day it all changed. The day I started to never take anything for granted. The day I learned to take charge of my life. It was the day I was diagnosed with cancer."

—Lance Armstrong

At age 25, Lance Armstrong was one of the world's best cyclists. He had won many championship titles including a cycling World Championship, multiple victories at the Tour du Pont, a spot on the 1996 United States Olympic team, and was closing in on the "Super Bowl" of bicycle racing, the Tour de France.

Then he learned the chronic pain he had long ignored was aggressive testicular cancer, and it had spread to his lungs and brain. Doctors put his chances of survival at less than 50%, seriously underestimating the young Texan's competitive spirit.

Armstrong swore he would be a cancer survivor, not a victim. "Anything is possible," he said. "You can be told you have a 90% chance, or a 50% chance, or a 1% chance. But you have to believe, and you have to fight."

Armstrong began his fight by learning about his disease and the treatment. Confident in his doctors' skills, he started a rigorous surgery and chemotherapy.

As he went through the treatment, he decided to use his experience to do something positive. Even before he knew he would survive, he founded The Lance Armstrong Foundation for cancer research and support programs for other cancer survivors.

Then he beat the cancer. The doctors said it was gone. Probably for life.

But the exhausting treatment program had sapped his strength and wasted his muscles. The dream of racing again in the Tour de France was alive, but it would take a grueling conditioning program and months of serious training. "Pain is temporary," Lance said. "It may last a minute, or an hour, or a day, or a year, but eventually it will subside and something else will take its place. If I quit, however, it lasts forever." That's the Armstrong Attitude.

In 1999, Lance took his place at the starting line in Paris for the 23-day, 1,800-mile race. When it ended, the winner's yellow jersey belonged to him. And that was just the beginning. Lance now has won the Tour de France a record seven consecutive times. Little wonder that yellow is the color of the 80 million Live Strong wristbands his foundation has sold in 60 countries. Perhaps you wear one.

Today, the Lance Armstrong Foundation raises money for research and programs to improve the lives of cancer survivors. It has committed more than $20 million in grants to community nonprofit organizations that serve the needs of people living with cancer. It offers grant recipients regular training and technical support.

In 2005, the Foundation gave $500,000 to cancer survivors affected by Hurricane Katrina.

In 2007, Lance, with Andre Agassi, Muhammad Ali, Warrick Dunn, Jeff Gordon, Mia Hamm, Tony Hawk, Andrea Jaeger, Jackie Joyner-Kersee, Mario Lemieux, Alonzo Mourning, and Cal Ripken Jr., started Athletes for Hope, an organization helping professional athletes become involved in charitable causes and to inspire non-athletes to volunteer and support their communities.

Lance Armstrong is a beacon of hope for everyone with a cancer diagnosis. He proved it can be beaten, and a person can be better for it. His proof? Seven yellow jerseys.

"Without cancer, I never would have won a single Tour de France," he said. "Cancer taught me a plan for more purposeful living, and that in turn taught me how to train and to win more purposefully.

It taught me that pain has a reason, and that sometimes the experience of losing things has its own value in the scheme of life. Pain and loss are great enhancers."

"Whatever you can do,
or dream you can,
begin it.
Boldness has genius, power and magic in it.
Begin it now."
—W. H. Murray

Kent Keith

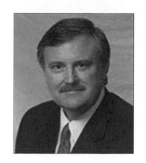

Do It Anyway

In 1966, Kent Keith was a high school senior in Honolulu, Hawaii. During that year, not only was he Student Body President at Roosevelt High School, he also established the Hawaii Student Leadership Institute, a summer workshop for high school student leaders. Against the backdrop of the tumultuous Sixties, student activism rocked even the tranquility of the island paradise. Keith steadfastly provided an alternative tone, encouraging students to care about each other and to achieve change by using the system, instead of fighting it.

From there he went to Harvard where, in his sophomore year, the 19-year-old started writing two small booklets for high school student leaders: "The Silent Revolution: Dynamic Leadership in the Student Council" (1968), and "The Silent Majority: The Problem of Apathy and the Student Council" (1971). In chapter two of one booklet, he included a piece called "Brotherly What?"—defining what he called the "Paradoxical Commandments." "I laid down these commandments as a challenge," Keith said. "The challenge is to always do what is right and good and true, no matter what, because if you don't, many of the things that need to be done in our world will never get done." This pamphlet became very popular among students.

Fast-forward 30 years and several paths—Rhodes Scholar, attorney, state government official, high-tech park developer, and university president— Kent Keith is now 55 and a senior executive for the Honolulu YMCA. He was attending a Rotary International Club meeting a couple of weeks after Mother Teresa's death when, in her honor, a fellow Rotarian shared a piece written by her as the "thought for the day." Kent listened to the poem, which started, "People are illogical, unreasonable and self-centered. Love them anyway." He recalled feeling "completely surreal" when, expecting to be moved by the words of the inimitable "Angel in Calcutta," he recognized words he had written 30 years before.

With a little research, Keith quickly found the biography, "Mother Teresa: A Simple Path" compiled by Lucinda Vardey. It contained eight of his 10 original Paradoxical Commandments, reformatted as a poem called "Anyway," with no author listed. The reference simply said it hung on the wall of Mother Teresa's children's home in Calcutta.

"It moved me so much that the commandments had wound up on Mother Teresa's wall," said Keith, who with his wife, Elizabeth, had adopted three children from orphanages in Japan and Romania. "I was deeply honored to have my words associated with Mother Teresa. I got the chills and felt like laughing and crying at the same time."

Curious to know more, Keith searched the Internet and was shocked to find thousands of references to his Paradoxical Commandments. They had been used in graduation speeches, sermons, and dozens of books—sometimes properly attributed to Keith, sometimes to Mother Teresa, sometimes simply cited as "anonymous." They'd even been attributed to rock star Ted Nugent. Unknown to Keith, his written words had been touching millions around the world for 30 years.

Keith is far more delighted with the impact and distribution of his words than bothered by inaccurate attribution. "While this expression of words and ideas may be mine, the concepts themselves are fundamental and universal. They are truths that make sense to almost everyone." Keith shared his spiritual journey in his two subsequent books, *Anyway: The Paradoxical Commandment* and *Do It Anyway*.

"The Paradoxical Commandments have a strong spiritual basis," Keith notes, "but I never wanted them to send a purely idealistic, 'safe in the garden' message. In *Do It Anyway*, I wanted to bring the Commandments down to earth and show how lots of people are living them on a daily basis, even in very difficult situations. I wanted to share the stories of people who are using these principles to break away from excuses and make the right decisions for the right reasons. To me, that is what is really inspiring."

The Paradoxical Commandments
...by Dr. Kent M. Keith

People are illogical, unreasonable, and self-centered.
Love them anyway.

If you do good, people will accuse you of selfish ulterior motives.
Do good anyway.

If you are successful, you win false friends and true enemies.
Succeed anyway.

The good you do today will be forgotten tomorrow.
Do good anyway.

Honesty and frankness make you vulnerable.
Be honest and frank anyway.

The biggest men and women with the biggest ideas can be shot down
by the smallest men and women with the smallest minds.
Think big anyway.

People favor underdogs but follow only top dogs.
Fight for a few underdogs anyway.

What you spend years building may be destroyed overnight.
Build anyway.

People really need help but may attack you if you do help them.
Help people anyway.

Give the world the best you have and you'll get kicked in the teeth.
Give the world the best you have anyway.

Conclusion

Postscript

The impact of *The Gift of Passionaries* will be measured by what it means to *you*, the reader: How will it affect your life? Which profiles ignited your own passions? Are you inspired to get involved? Each one of us can make a difference, and those differences ripple out and change the world.

"The gift" of this book is three-fold: First, the gift shows what is being done for those in need by passionaries. Second, the gift shows how the world is positively blessed by creative-thinkers with new ideas for solving social problems. Finally, the gift demonstrates how passionaries model and mentor giving to others. For all those who give, especially passionaries, donors, and volunteers: **Thank you!** You make this country and our world great.

Throughout the years of putting this book together, the "how in the world did something like this ever get started and grow?" aspect of each nonprofit has fascinated me. While this is not a "how-to" book, there is a common thread in the nature of passionaries: Someone is challenged by adversity, there is a moment in time—a "click" when passion connects with an idea and the "I can do that" is voiced. The lights come on, momentum builds, often others come alongside, miracles happen, and lives are changed.

As I've chronicled these miracle-makers and their passionate adventures, I feel incredibly blessed and inspired. These stories of courage inspire change. However, like the countless points of light we see in a starry night sky, there are endless passionaries yet to profile. With over 1 million known nonprofits, just listing the organizations' names would fill volumes of books.

This is the second in my *Passionaries* collection. Future volumes are under way and will come out one or two times a year.

A few of the remarkable profiles earmarked for the next book are:

- ♥ Robert Macauley (AmeriCares)
- ♥ Wess Stafford (Compassion International)
- ♥ Merilee Pierce Dunker (World Vision)
- ♥ Jason Russell (Invisible Children)
- ♥ John Walsh (National Center for Missing & Exploited Children)
- ♥ Eunice Kennedy Shriver (Special Olympics)
- ♥ Darrell Scott (Rachel's Challenge)

I hope that at least one profile in this volume will inspire you to find a cause you are passionate about and join in. There are three ways you can join the efforts to make a difference:

- ♥ Start an organization like the passionaries profiled in this book.
- ♥ Work with others who share your passion to build momentum for a cause.
- ♥ Join one of the organizations mentioned in this book using the contact information provided at the end of each profile and in this appendix, or join any other organization that inspires you.
- ♥ Become a Passionor—donate.

We are surrounded by goodness, and we have the opportunity, and the privilege, of passing this goodness on to friends and family who share our desire to make the world a better place. You cannot begin to imagine what passion you may spark or how many lives your sparks might touch. I pass these stories on to you in the hope it will spark a passion in your life that will ripple out to many others.

Passion breeds enthusiasm—one of the most powerful engines of success. When passionaries take action, they do it with all their might and soul. They are focused, energetic, and faithful. As Ralph Waldo Emerson once said, "Nothing great was ever achieved without enthusiasm."

What are you going to do with the information in these profiles? It is your life and your choice. As these stories show, you also have the power to change the world. Find your own passion. Start, build, join or donate—do something. Make a difference for others. Passionate!

The Passionaries Project

If you have been touched by this book and want to help make it available to others, we invite you to participate in The Passionaries Project. A team of passionaries' fans who have been inspired by this book are convinced it deserves a reading across the length and breadth of our country. Not only are these profiles compelling, but the book has a literary quality that sets it apart as a special gift for you to give those who have made a difference in your life.

Producers are working to create a television show featuring passionaries, and getting a sufficient number of these books out in circulation will go a long way toward making this a reality. Many in the media know there is a need for positive television that reflects our true values, and the timing is ripe. Word of mouth is still the most effective tool to help this book gain traction in our culture. We each need to spread the word.

If you are moved by the message of *The Gift of Passionaries*, you may already have some unique ideas about how you can tell others about it. Here are some ideas to help you share this book with others:

- ♥ Give the book to friends, family, mentors, passionaries, teachers, even strangers, as a gift. They not only get a compelling, page-turning book, but also a magnificent "thank you" or an encouragement to make a difference in the world.

- ♥ Share how this book has affected your life on e-mail lists, blogs you frequent, and other places you interact with people on the Internet. Link them to our website. If you have a website or a blog, consider sharing a bit about this book and how it touched your life. You can recommend it and link others to our website, www.passionaries.com.

- ♥ Write a book review for your favorite magazine or local newspaper. Ask your preferred radio show or local television station to invite the author to be a guest. Media people often consider the requests of their listeners more seriously than press releases from publicists.

- ♥ If you are in a book club, recommend *The Gift of Passionaries* then have a passion-filled discussion about which profiles touched you the most. Sample questions for book club discussions can be found on our website. And if you write to the author through the website, she will do her best to call in and participate in your discussion.

- ♥ If you are a business or nonprofit leader or are involved in a foundation, consider giving this book as a gift to your board members and leaders in your organization. It makes a great Christmas gift or year-end "thank you."

- ♥ If you own a retail business, consider putting this book on your counter display to sell to customers. Books are available at a discounted rate for resale. Individuals can receive a volume discount price for orders of eight books or more.

- ♥ Consider buying a set of books for your local school, hospital, women's shelter, prison, or your favorite nonprofit outreach so people there can be empowered by the profiles.

For more up-to-date ideas and information on how you can help, please check out The Passionaries Project on our website:

www.passionaries.com

You can also apply for the $300 stipend offered through our website by writing a profile that might be chosen for use in future books. Write stories about passionaries you know, and help celebrate high-impact, financially-efficient, volunteer-friendly, eclectic, and interesting nonprofit organizations that have been started within the past 30 years.

Service Groups in the United States

One way to get involved in volunteering is through your local church or synagogue; another is to join an organization already making a difference in your community and around the world. The following is a list of organizations that are recommended as the easiest, most fun, and widely educational ways to volunteer. Check them out!

Elks ≈ Founded in 1868, The Benevolent and Protective Order of Elks is dedicated to charitable works and is the largest *fraternal* organization in our nation with more than 2,000 lodges made up of well over 1.25 million members. Members are patriotic Americans who believe in God (nondenominational), want to be an active force for good in their community, want to be better citizens, and enjoy the good fellowship of enthusiastic, successful men.

Elks stage year-round shows and entertainments for disabled veterans in every Veterans Administration (VA) hospital in the country. Elks donated the first VA hospital to the United States government and pioneered the observance of June 14 as Flag Day, the anniversary of Old Glory's birth in 1777.

Since the group's inception, the Elks have contributed more than $333 million dollars for charitable, welfare, and patriotic programs. The Elks are second only to the United States government in the amount of money provided for scholarships each year. Elks scholarships are measured in the millions of dollars annually. They sponsor many youth groups—sports, scouting, and 4-H clubs, D.A.R.E. programs, summer camps, adopt-a-school, Hoop Shoot, etc.

The Elks do not compete with other civic organizations. They recognize the philanthropic efforts of many other civic and community groups, assisting those organizations when and where possible. The Elks motto is: "The faults of our brothers we write upon the sand, their virtues upon the tablets of love and memory."

The Elks National Headquarters
2750 N. Lakeview Avenue
Chicago, Illinois 60614-1889
Phone: (773) 755-4700
E-mail: ElksOnline@aol.com
Website: www.elks.org

Jaycees ≈ The Jaycees have been an important force for good in America and around the world for more than 85 years through men and women ages 18 to 40. Jaycees gives members the tools and training to be successful in business development, management, community service, and international endeavors. It provides leadership and direction to communities, states, and nations worldwide, with its members investing their time and energy in civic affairs.

Nationwide, 4,300 Jaycee chapters have 200,000 members and range in size from 20 to more than 1,000 members. Jaycees helped establish AirMail services in America with Jaycee Charles Lindbergh, and have raised millions of dollars for causes such as the Muscular Dystrophy Association and the March of Dimes. They have built parks, playgrounds, hospitals, ball fields, and housing for the elderly while conducting service and support programs in thousands of communities nationwide.

Jaycees can be found in all walks of life: government leaders such as past Presidents Bill Clinton and Gerald Ford, business tycoons such as Domino's Pizza mogul Tom Monaghan, registered nurse and former Miss America Kaye Lani Rae Rafko-Wilson, and sports heroes like basketball great Larry Bird. Name the field and Jaycees can be found at the forefront.

With the nation's focus on volunteerism, from the smallest towns to the largest cities, the Jaycees are enlarging areas of opportunity for young people.

The Jaycees National Service Center

Phone: (800) JAYCEES

Website: www.usjaycees.org

Support the goals and objectives of Jaycees through corporate partnerships or membership benefits directly aimed at this proactive market. Contact USJC's resource development manager at (918) 584-2481 ext. 412.

Kiwanis (also: Keys and Builders Club) ≈ Kiwanis is a worldwide club for community leader volunteers dedicated to changing the world, one child and one community at a time. Kiwanis offers an opportunity for service and fun while improving the community, the nation, and the world through service and fellowship in friendships that are sincere and lasting.

Founded in 1915, Kiwanis and its service leadership programs now boast a membership of more than 600,000 men, women, and youth in nearly 16,000 clubs in more than 70 countries and geographic areas. Kiwanians have volunteered more than 21 million hours and invested more than $113 million in communities around the world.

Kiwanis continues its service emphasis of "Young Children: Priority One," which focuses on the special needs of children from prenatal development to age 5. In a typical year, "Young Children: Priority One" service projects involve more than 14 million dollars and 1 million volunteer hours. In 1994, Kiwanis launched its first worldwide service project, a successful $75 million campaign in partnership with UNICEF to significantly diminish iodine deficiency disorders (IDD) by the year 2000. IDD projects have been funded in 95 nations. Kiwanis International Foundation has raised nearly $100 million to eliminate IDD worldwide.

Kiwanis International is the only service organization that builds leaders at every level—from the youngest Kiwanis Kids all the way through several youth and adult programs, including:

- ♥ **Circle Kiwanis International (CKI):** on 550 college and university campuses
- ♥ **Key Leaders:** a new leadership experience for exceptional leaders from 8th to 12th grades
- ♥ **Key Club:** 245,000 high school service leaders working on a variety of social causes
- ♥ **Builder's Club:** 40,000 middle and high school students implement service-learning principles
- ♥ **K-Kids:** service clubs for elementary students, teaching the value of helping others

- ♥ **Terrific Kids:** recognizing character with prizes for "Thoughtful, Enthusiastic, Respectful, Responsible, Inclusive, Friendly, Inquisitive, Capable kids.

- ♥ **BUG - Bringing Up Grades:** recognizes students who improve their grades

- ♥ **AKTION:** 200 clubs allow adults with disabilities to serve with initiative and leadership skills

"Young Children: Priority One" is the Kiwanis program focusing on the needs of children in areas of pediatric trauma, safety, child care, early development, infant health, nutrition, and parenting skills. The typical Kiwanis club plans numerous projects each year that focus on special needs in a community. They include fighting substance abuse, promoting literacy, supporting youth sports, and other projects involving children or people in need. In high schools and colleges, Key Club and Circle K are the largest service organizations of their kind. Each meeting is guaranteed to engender fun, service, and camaraderie. Get involved:

Kiwanis International

3636 Woodview Trace

Indianapolis, Indiana 46268

Phone: (800) KIWANIS

Website: www.kiwanisone.org

Lions ≈ The International Association of Lions Clubs was created in 1917 by Chicago businessman Melvin Jones. Today it is the largest service organization in the world, with over 1.3 million members in more than 42,000 clubs in 202 countries. Lions took up sight conservation as their major goal after Helen Keller spoke at the Lions International Convention at Cedar Point, Ohio, in 1925. Members conduct vision and health screenings, support eye hospitals, award scholarships, assist youth, provide help in times of disaster, build parks, and much more.

Lions clubs are service clubs with social benefits, where members focus on health, primarily sight conservation, although other projects are pursued such as drug awareness programs in high schools, diabetes awareness programs, and other programs specific to individual clubs and districts. For example, Massachusetts Lions created an eye research fund that gives research grants to Massachusetts universities and hospitals and has given more than $12 million in research grants since its inception. The Kentucky Lions have built and financially support an eye hospital.

In 1990, Lions launched its most aggressive sight preservation effort, SightFirst. The $202 million program strives to rid the world of preventable and reversible blindness by supporting desperately needed health care services. Lions' work in the area of sight conservation is carried out at many levels. Individual clubs sponsor free eye screening programs using mobile eye clinics. In many countries, clubs sponsor camps where cataract surgeries are performed at no charge for people who can't afford medical treatment. Many clubs in the United States collect old eyeglasses for distribution to people in need in other countries. Lions' services to humanity range from purchasing eyeglasses for a child whose parents can't afford them to multimillion dollar programs to cure blindness on a worldwide scale.

In addition to sight programs, Lions Clubs International is committed to providing services for youth. Lions clubs also work to improve the environment, build homes for the disabled, support diabetes education, conduct hearing programs and, through their foundation, provide disaster relief around the world.

The Lions Clubs International
300 22nd Street
Oak Brook, Illinois 90521
Phone: (708) 571-5466
Website: www.lionsclubs.org

Optimist International ≈ Meeting the needs of young people in communities worldwide, Optimist Clubs have been "Bringing Out the Best in Kids" since 1919. Optimist Clubs conduct positive service projects aimed at providing a helping hand to youth. Club members are best known in their communities for their upbeat attitudes. By believing in young people and empowering them to be the best they can be, Optimist volunteers continually make the world a better place to live. There are 101,000 individual volunteer members in more than 3,200 autonomous clubs. Optimists conduct 65,000 service projects each year, serving 6 million young people. Optimists also spend $78 million on their communities annually.

Optimists believe in positive thinking as a philosophy of life, utilizing the tenets of the Optimist Creed: to promote an active interest in good government and civic affairs; to inspire respect for the law; to promote patriotism and work for international accord and friendship among all people; to aid and encourage the development of youth, in the belief that the giving of one's self in service to others will advance the well-being of humankind, community life, and the world.

The Optimist Creed
Promise yourself –
To be so strong that nothing can disturb your peace of mind.
To talk health, happiness, and prosperity to every person you meet.
To make all your friends feel that there is something in them.
To look at the sunny side of everything and
make your optimism come true.
To think only of the best, to work only for the best,
and to expect only the best.
To be just as enthusiastic about the success of others
as you are about your own.
To forget the mistakes of the past and press on to
the greater achievements of the future.
To wear a cheerful countenance at all times and
give every living creature you meet a smile.
To give so much time to the improvement of yourself
that you have no time to criticize others.
To be too large for worry, too noble for anger, too strong for fear,
and too happy to permit the presence of trouble.
– authored by Christian D. Larson, 1912

A major focus of Optimist International today is drug abuse prevention. Optimist Clubs sponsor "Just Say No" clubs and many other types of activities that educate youth about drugs and support a drug-free lifestyle. Since 1928, Optimist International has sponsored their annual Oratorical Contest for youth. Today, more than $150,000 in scholarships is awarded each year to contest winners. Optimist International also sponsors the largest international golf tournament for young people, the Optimist Junior World Championships. Other major Optimist programs include the Optimist Essay Contest, Optimist Youth Appreciation, Optimist Bike Safety Week, and Optimist Respect for Law Week.

Have fun, be optimistic, and make a difference for kids.

To find an Optimist Club in your area, go to www.optimist.org.

Rotary ≈ A young lawyer named Paul P. Harris founded the first Rotary Club in Chicago, Illinois, in 1905 when he gathered in friendship a group of young men, each engaged in a different form of service to the public. That basis for membership—one person from each business and profession in the community—still exists today. At first, the members of the new club met in rotation at their various places of business, and this suggested the name "Rotary."

Rotary has grown into a worldwide organization of more than 1.2 million business, professional, and community leaders. Members of Rotary Clubs, known as Rotarians, provide humanitarian service, encourage high ethical standards in all vocations, and help build goodwill and peace in the world. There are more than 32,000 Rotary Clubs in more than 200 countries and geographical areas. Clubs are nonpolitical, nonreligious, and open to all cultures, races, and creeds.

As signified by the motto "Service Above Self," Rotary's main objective is service—in the community, in the workplace, and throughout the world. Since 1947, Rotarians have contributed more than $1.9 billion to The Rotary Foundation. Rotary clubs everywhere have one basic ideal: the "Ideal of Service," which is thoughtfulness of and helpfulness to others.

In the 1980s, when 1,000 children were infected by polio every day in 125 countries, Rotary made a major commitment to rid the world of the disease. Since that time, Rotary has helped immunize 2 billion children—5 million have been spared disability, and more than 250,000 deaths have been prevented. By 2006, polio cases declined by 99 percent, with fewer than 2,000 cases reported. Yet many people still live under the threat of polio, which is why Rotary and its global partners are committed to a new goal of reaching every child with the vaccine and eliminating this disease worldwide.

There are almost as many world-changing Rotary projects as there are clubs. Rotarians embody and enable friendship, fun, joint commitment to service, and community building. Youth outreaches include:

- ♥ Rotary Youth Leadership Awards (RYLA) for youth service with compatible age ranges
- ♥ Rotaract: a Rotary-sponsored service club for young men and women ages 18 to 30 with 7,000 clubs in 163 countries
- ♥ Interact: Rotary's service club for youth aged 14 to 18—really fun and active
- ♥ Rotary Youth Exchange: each year, 8,000 students spend up to a year living with host families and attending school in a different country

Rotary International, World Headquarters
One Rotary Center
560 Sherman Ave.
Evanston, Illinois 60201
Phone: (708) 866-3000, FAX: (708) 328-8554
Website: www.rotary.org

Soroptimist ≈ Soroptimist is an international service organization for business and professional women who work to improve the lives of women and girls. Almost 95,000 Soroptimists in about 120 countries and territories contribute time, service, and financial support to community-based and international projects that benefit women and girls.

The name, Soroptimist, means "best for women," and that's what the organization strives to achieve. They represent women at their best, working to help other women be their best.

Soroptimist members belong to local clubs, which determine the focus of volunteer work in their communities. Club projects range from renovating domestic violence shelters and providing mammograms to low-income women to sponsoring self-esteem workshops for teenage girls. In addition, Soroptimists participate in organization-wide programs, including the Soroptimist Women's Opportunity Awards, Soroptimist Club Grants for Women and Girls, the Soroptimist Workplace Campaign to End Domestic Violence, the Soroptimist Making a Difference for Women Award, the Soroptimist Violet Richardson Award, and Soroptimists STOP Trafficking. Clubs also participate in the "Live Your Dream" campaign, which encourages all women to live their dreams while helping others do the same.

Soroptimist International of the Americas
Two Penn Center Plaza, Suite 1000
Philadelphia, Pennsylvania 19102
Phone: (800) 942-4629
Website: www.soroptimist.org

"Earth's crammed with heaven,
And every common bush afire with God.
But only he who sees takes off his shoes;
The rest sit round it and pluck blackberries."
—Elizabeth Barrett Browning

The Legacy of Saint Francis of Assisi ≈ Born in the Italian town of Assisi, Italy, in 1182, Francis was the good-looking son of the wealthy merchant Bernadone. Francis was brought up surrounded by luxury, love, laughter, and many friends, including the children of noble men.

Being soft-hearted and compassionate, Francis gave much of his money to the poor—much to the displeasure of his father. When a serious disease threatened his life, he was saved by a heavenly miracle. Seeing a vision of the Lord, Francis renounced his old ways of living and gave himself to a life of purity dedicated to serving humanity.

Shunned by his angry father and noble friends, Francis left his home and lived in a mountain cave near Assisi, wearing a coarse dress and eating simple food. He was humble and loved all of God's creatures. Twelve people were so attracted by his saintliness that they gave all their wealth to the poor, and followed Francis.

Francis' gospel of kindness and love spread throughout Europe, and he formed the Order of Franciscans, who take a vow of poverty, chastity, love, and obedience. Saint Francis was known as the little poor man of Assisi, and the prayer that he left behind has touched every generation since his death in 1228. The Prayer of Saint Francis is a blueprint on which we all can pattern our lives, thoughts, and actions.

The Prayer of Saint Francis

"O Lord, make me an instrument of Thy Peace!
Where there is hatred, let me sow love;
Where there is injury, pardon;
Where there is discord, harmony;
Where there is doubt, faith;
Where there is despair, hope;
Where there is darkness, light, and
Where there is sorrow, joy.
Oh Divine Master, grant that I may not
so much seek to be consoled as to console;
to be understood as to understand; to be loved
as to love; for it is in giving that we receive;
It is in pardoning that we are pardoned;
and it is in dying that we are born to Eternal Life."

Acknowledgments

My immense gratitude also goes to a personal hero of mine, Dr. Chuck Colson for writing the introduction. You have made and continue to make indelible marks on the world. And a huge "thank you" hug goes to the friends who have endorsed this book. You have all been an encouraging and important part of *The Gift of Passionaries*.

Thank you to the professionals who have helped mold this book. Abundant appreciation and heartfelt thanks to Jan Funchess, Manda Gibson, Teri Haymaker, Ron Humphrey, Don Ingel, and Mark Kelly for fabulous editing; my agent Ellen Stiefler for remarkable legal and marketing advice; Rodney Bissell, Jan Funchess, Ellen Goodwin, Teri Haymaker, and Gary Johns for great graphic design; and Sivia Finn and Lisa Frost for being my friends and webmasters.

When we venture into uncharted waters, as I have with these passionaries books, we are given what I call "earth angels" to help guide us toward safe port. I am very fortunate and grateful to the individuals who have helped me in oh-so-many ways on this project. First, to my family—Denny, Erin, David, Kersten, and Douglas—and then to supportive friends who have helped this passionary movement, especially Ellen Stiefler, George Francis, Susan McClellan, Cinda Lucas, Tom Sullivan, Art Ulene, Bettie Youngs, Brendon Buchard, Matthew Bennett, Scott Evans, Paul Pickard, Ron and Mary Jenson, Steve Harrison, Jack and Pima Templeton, Muriel Nellis, and Linda and Phil Lader. Your fingerprints are all over this book because of your love and support.

Appendix

Selected and Suggested Readings and Movies

Books

Audio Adrenaline. *The Hands and Feet Project*. Ventura, California: Regal Books, 2006.

Attwood, Janet Bray and Chris Attwood. *The Passion Test: The Effortless Path to Discovering Your Destiny*. New York, New York: Hudson Street Press, 2006, 2007.

Behring, Ken. *Road to Purpose: One Man's Journey Bringing Hope to Millions*. Alexandria, Virginia: Blackhawk Press, VSP Books, 2004.

Graham, Franklin. *Rebel With A Cause*. Nashville, Tennessee: Thomas Nelson, 1997.

Haugen, Gary A. *Good News About Justice: A Witness of Courage in a Hurting World*. Downers Grove, Illinois: Inter Varsity Press, 1999.

Hunter, Zach. *Be the Change: Your Guide to Freeing Slaves and Changing the World*. Grand Rapids, Michigan: Zondervan, 2007.

Keith, Kent. *Anyway: The Paradoxical Commandments: Finding Personal Meaning in a Crazy World*. New York, New York: Penguin Putman, Inc., 2001.

Kidder, Tracy. *Mountains Beyond Mountains*. New York, New York: Random House, Inc., 2004.

Krabacher, Susie Scott. *Angels of a Lower Flight: One Woman's Mission To Save A Country... One Child at a Time*. New York, New York: Touchstone/ Simon & Schuster, 2007.

Nunn, Michelle. *Be The Change: Change the World. Change Yourself*. Atlanta, Georgia: Hundreds of Heads Books, LLC, 2006.

Schuller, Robert A. *Walking in Your Own Shoes*. New York, New York: Faith Words, 2007.

Vitale, Dick with Dick Weiss. *Dick Vitale: Living a Dream*. Champaign, Illinois: Sports Publishing LLC, 2003.

Movies on Passionary Themes

Amazing Grace. Director: Michael Apted, writer (WGA): Steven Knight. FourBoys Films, Walden Media, 2007

John Adams. With Paul Giamatti and Laura Linney, HBO Films, 2008.

Pay It Forward. Director: Mimi Leder, writers (WGA): Leslie Dixon (screenplay), Catherine Ryan Hyde (book), Warner Brothers, 2000.

Freedom Writers. Director: Richard LaGravenese. With Hilary Swank and Patrick Dempsey, writers (WGA): Richard LaGravenese (screenplay), Erin Gruwell and The Freedom Writers (book), Paramount Pictures, 2006.

> *"I dream...*
> *I test my dreams*
> *against my beliefs,*
> *I dare to take risks,*
> *and I execute my vision*
> *to make those dreams come true."*
> *—Walt Disney*

Web Sites for Rating Financial Efficiency of Nonprofit Organizations

♥ Better Business Bureau's Wise Giving Alliance: www.give.org

♥ Charity Navigator: www.charitynavigator.org

♥ Oprah (recommends some terrific Oprah-rated nonprofits): www.oprah.com

♥ Peter Drucker Foundation, Leader to Leader Institute: www.pfdf.org

♥ Guide Star provides information to make better decisions, and encourages charitable giving: www.guidestar.org

Web Sites for Direct On-Line Giving

DonorsChoose: www.donorschoose.org (New York). Founded in 2000, they connect donors directly to classroom projects in public schools.

GlobalGiving: www.globalgiving.com (Washington). Founded in 2000, this site allows donors to support international charitable causes.

Kiva: www.kiva.org (San Francisco). Founded in 2005, Kiva allows people to lend funds at 0% interest to entrepreneurs in developing countries.

Modest Needs: www.modestneeds.org (New York). Founded in 2002, this site allows people to make donations to low-income individuals who need short-term help.

OptINnow: www.optinnow.org (Chicago). Founded in 2008 by Opportunity International, this site permits the choice of a third-country individual in need of a small microcredit loan to create a business. This mini-amount maximizes entrepreneurship.

Web Sites for Volunteer Opportunities in your area:

♥ www.passionaries.com

♥ www.1-800-volunteer.org

Notes

The information for the profiles in *The Gift of Passionaries* came from personal interviews and the passionaries' cited websites.

Susan Corrigan and Betty Mohlenbrach stories have been updated from their original publication in *Passionaries™: Turning Compassion into Action*, Barbara Metzler. Templeton Foundation Press, 2006, Susan Corrigan (page 22) and Betty Mohlenbrock (page 174).

All information for the following stories was taken directly from their respective web sites:

Lance Armstrong, LiveStrong

Tiger Woods, Tiger Foundation

For further selected readings on these profiles, see the following:

Endnotes

[1]Giving USA, a publication of the Giving USA Foundation™, researched and written by the Center on Philanthropy at Indiana University, 14–17.

[2]Di Mento, Maria & Lewis, Nicole 2008. *A big year for giving*, The Chronicle of Philanthropy, volume XX, No. 7, 7–10.

[3]Giving USA, a publication of the Giving USA Foundation™, researched and written by the Center on Philanthropy at Indiana University, 27, 34.

[4]Jensen, Brennen 2008. Giving by family foundations jumps 21%, study finds. The Chronicle of Philanthropy. volume XX, No. 12, 16.

[5]Barton, Noelle; Preston, Caroline; Wilhelm, Ian 2006. Slow growth at the biggest foundations. The Chronicle of Philanthropy. volume XVIII, No. 11, 14.

[6]Giving USA, a publication of the Giving USA Foundation™, researched and written by the Center on Philanthropy at Indiana University, 28, 31.

[7]Cohen, Todd 2007, *Corporate foundations give over $4 billion.* Philanthropy Journal, http://www.philanthropyjournal.org/archive/132315. And Austin, Algernon: Asstistant Director at the Foundation Center 2007. Key facts on corporate foundations / May 2007, the Foundation Center. New York, NY, http://foundationcenter.org/gainknowledge/research/pdf/keyfacts_corp_2007.pdf.

[8]Barton, Noellle & Preston, Caroline 2008. *Overseas giving by American companies is on the rise.* The Chronicle of Philanthropy, volume XX, No. 21, 7.

[9]The Index of Global Philanthropy 2007, a publication of the Hudson Institute, researched and written by The Index of Global Philanthropy Team, 2, 6-11.

[10]Preston, Caroline 2008. *Number of Americans who volunteer rises, survey finds.* The Chronicle of Philanthropy, volume XX, No. 11, 27.

[11]The Index of Global Philanthropy 2007. a publication of the Hudson Institute, researched and written by The Index of Global Philanthropy Team, 21.

[12]Giving USA, a publication of the Giving USA Foundation™, researched and written by the Center on Philanthropy at Indiana University, 45.

[13]Barton, Noelle & Schwinn, Elizabeth 2007. *Modest gains in giving. The Philanthropy 400.* The Chronicle of Philanthropy, volume XX, No. 2, 40.

Index

LOOK FOR

THE NEXT BOOK FROM

BARBARA METZLER

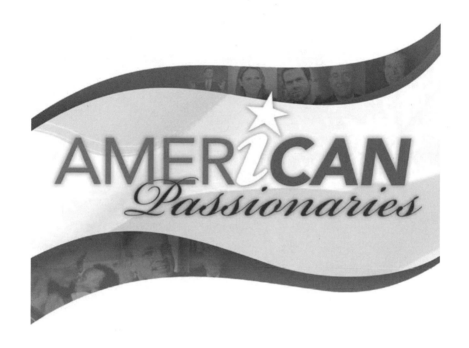

COMING WINTER 2009

Enjoy inspiration and possibilities...

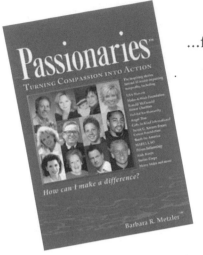

...from Barbara Metzler's
first book...

Filled with stories about real-life heroes like:

- ♥ Mary Kay Beard, founder and president of Angel Tree Project
- ♥ Jimmy Murray, founder of Ronald McDonald Houses
- ♥ Millard Fuller, founder of Habitat for Humanity
- ♥ Stan Curtis, founder and president of USA Harvest
- ♥ Wendy Kopp, founder and president of Teach for America
- ♥ Don Stephens, founder and president of Mercy Ships

And so many more...*Passionaries* will fill your heart with hope and the potential of American hearts and show you how you too can make a difference.

For bulk orders or questions visit our website at passionaries.com.

Praise for The Gift of Passionaries

"Each of the profiles in this inspiring book is food for our hungry hearts. Savor the stories and share them with family and friends."
—Stan Curtis, Founder and CEO of USA Harvest

"For people wanting to change the world... *The Gift of Passionaries* provides an invaluable road map. Way to go!" — Michael Davidson, CEO, Gen Next

"Metzler has given us an inspiring and powerful collection of extra-ordinary forces at work in the hearts of good people. They teach us how sacrifice is turned to potential and deep meaning comes from giving. These stories push us to ask, 'What can I do?'"
— Max De Pree, Chairman of Herman Miller,
author of "Leadership is an Art"

"Passionaries helps us never have to say again; 'evil exists when good people do nothing.' It's what television shows need to be all about... This book is an empowering gift for anyone wanting to find your mission and purpose in life."
—Ken Ferguson, CEO Mpower Media, movie producer of "Bella"

"Barbara Metzler has done it again! Read one or two of these moving stories each night and be inspired. These passionaries will renew your hope for the world!"
—Millard Fuller, Passionary Founder and President of Habitat for Humanity;
Founder and President of The Fuller Center for Housing

"This book is a 'gift' to anyone searching for role-models of compassion."
—U.S. Ambassador Tony P. Hall, former U.S. Ambassador
to Rome, Congressman, and Three-time Nobel Peace Prize Nominee

"We saw 'ginormous' in the dictionary. 'Passionary' should be next. It's where our hearts should be."
—Nicole Lapin, CNN Anchor at the Leaders of NOW Conference,
Atlanta 2008, host of CNN's the Leaders of NOW

"The field of corporate philanthropy has become increasingly sophisticated. The social need for corporate community investment and the business case for giving, notwithstanding a challenging economic environment, are both growing exponentially. Barbara Metzler's new book on the role of Passionaries provides new insight in how business leaders can make a difference."
—Charles H. Moore, Executive Director,
Committee Encouraging Corporate Philanthropy

"This book's gift to you is the magic of passion which can ignite your heart to BE THE CHANGE. The inspiring passionaries profiled will enable you to change the world and change yourself."
—Michelle Nunn, Founder and President of
HandsOn Network/Points of Light Institute

"Exercise your soul and ignite your passion with this inspiring book. *The Gift of Passionaries* is sure to move you."
—Judi Sheppard Missett, Founder and CEO, Jazzercise International

"In sharing these remarkable stories, Barbara confirms for readers that one person really can make a difference. Like Barbara, this book is genuinely inspiring."
—Bobbi DePorter, President, Quantum Learning Network/
SuperCamp, author of "Quantum Success"

"Passion is the fuel that powers truly great organizations. Don't miss this important book that will inspire you to new heights of service to others."
—Rob Parker, CEO, Kiwanis International

"After you have read 'The Gift of Passionaries,' you will want to read it over and over again. It will inspire your soul."
—Lynne Twist, President, Soul of Money Institute, and
author of "Soul of Money." Co-founder of The Pachamama Alliance

"Here's a great book for soul nurture... Set this little gem up right next to your morning newspaper...and be reminded that there's an army of ordinary people doing extraordinary things to bring light in places of unthinkable darkness."
—Peggy Wehmeyer, former ABC News correspondent,
host and managing editor of "The World Vision Report"

"Passionaries taps into what makes Americans great and gives hope that each of us can make a difference. May these profiles circle the world!"
—Rev. Robert A. Schuller, Senior Pastor, Crystal Cathedral

"Barbara Metzler has done it again—bringing together stories of people who have discovered their God-given passion in life and are changing the world, one life at a time."
—Eric Swanson, Director of the Leadership Network

"The power and generosity of business leaders to positively change the world is captivatingly captured in this must read book. As a fellow member of World Presidents Organization, we thank you for the gift of these profiles, Barbara."
—Mark Van Ness, Vice Chairman of the Social Enterprise Networks for Young
Presidents Organization and World President's Organization